PA

D0265347

£6.50.

2

PERIPHERAL VASCULAR DISEASES:

Diagnosis and Management

Peripheral Vascular Diseases

DIAGNOSIS AND MANAGEMENT

H. Edward Holling
M.D., F.R.C.P., F.A.C.P.

*Associate Professor of Medicine and Chief of Vascular Service
of the Hospital of the University of Pennsylvania, Philadelphia
Formerly of the Scientific Staff of the British Medical Research
Council at Guy's Hospital, London*

PADDINGTON TECHNICAL
LIBRARY,
PADDINGTON GREEN,
LONDON. W2

J. B. Lippincott Company
Philadelphia • Toronto

PADDINGTON TECHNICAL
COLLEGE LIBRARY.

Date Y . 6. 74

21359

Acc. o. ... REFERENCE

Class No. 616·131

Copyright © 1972 by J. B. Lippincott Company
*This book is fully protected by copyright and, with the exception
of brief excerpts for review, no part of it may be reproduced in any
form by print, photoprint, microfilm or any other means without
written permission from the publisher.*

Distributed in Great Britain by
Blackwell Scientific Publications, Oxford, London, and Edinburgh

ISBN 0-397-50304-0
Library of Congress Catalog Card Number 72-4630
Printed in the United States of America
1 3 4 2

Library of Congress Cataloging in Publication Data

Holling, H   Edward.
   Peripheral vascular diseases.

   Includes bibliographies.
    1. Peripheral vascular diseases. I. Title. [DNLM:
1. Vascular diseases—Diagnoses. 2. Vascular diseases
—Therapy. WG 500 H741p 1972]
RC694.H64   616.1'31   72-4630
ISBN 0-397-50304-0

Preface

Almost 40 years ago Sir Thomas Lewis wrote an account of *Vascular Disorders of the Limbs* for the benefit of practitioners and students. At that time the study of the peripheral circulation appeared to be particularly suited to the application of scientific principles so that the knowledge gained could be applied to better understanding and management of vascular disorders. Sir Thomas' faith in this approach, which he called clinical science, was brilliantly displayed in his slim volume, and the ideas expressed in it are still basic to our understanding of disorders of the peripheral circulation.

Sir Thomas wrote after an era in which emphasis had been placed on practice rather than on investigation, and his purpose was to show how the care of patients with vascular disease could be improved if the scientific principles underlying their disorders were understood and applied. That ideal remains, though perhaps there is less reason to stress it now, for it is generally accepted. Emphasis now is tending back to the patient himself, and I trust that the chapters of this book will present the subject of vascular disease to students and practitioners in such a manner that patients may be cared for with better understanding of their condition.

In the past 40 years the spectrum of vascular diseases has changed. As always atherosclerosis obliterans is the most frequently encountered arterial disease. Aneurysm of the first part of the aorta due to syphilis has almost disappeared, but the number of cases of aneurysm of the abdominal aorta increases yearly. Thromboangiitis obliterans is fast disappearing, and the incidence of arteritis of other kinds is increasing. Treatment has been transformed. Arterial surgery has progressed from a rare surgical venture to a point where competence in vascular surgery can be expected of every good surgeon; and the physician must keep himself aware of progress in surgery in order to be able to give informed advice to his patients. Looking further ahead, there is reason to hope that the better understanding we have gained of the causes and effects of hyperlipoproteinemia will result in slowing the onslaught of atherosclerosis. The progress of treatment by drugs has been too long diverted by the quest for a vasodilator drug, when what is required is the means to attack the disease itself rather than its effect on blood vessels.

In writing this book I have not attempted to be encyclopedic but have given references to fuller accounts. I have stressed those aspects of vascular disorders which most often concern the physician in his care of patients. This is a personal account and is presented with the same caution with which Gilbert White presented his observations on the natural history of his parish of Selborne in 1765: "These observations are, I trust, true in the whole, though I do not pretend to show that they are perfectly void of mistake, or that a nice observer might not make many additions, since subjects of this kind are inexhaustible."

Contents

PART III
DISORDERS OF SMALL VESSELS

PART IV
DISORDERS OF VEINS AND LYMPHATICS

To my mentors

HUGH MONTGOMERY
RONALD T. GRANT
and
BROOKE ROBERTS

Part I

GENERAL TOPICS

1

The Peripheral Circulation

William Harvey conjectured that the arteries and veins must have "secret" anastomoses between them, and when the microscope revealed the secret of the capillaries it became customary to think of the peripheral circulation in terms of arteries, capillaries, and veins. With our present knowledge it is more informative to group the vessels into five categories. These are (1) the aorta and large arteries, which constitute a distribution system, (2) the arterioles, sometimes called the resistance vessels, which act as a regulatory system, (3) the microcirculation in which metabolites pass to and from the tissues across the endothelium, (4) a collecting system of veins carrying blood to the heart, and (5) the larger veins acting as a storage system.

THE DISTRIBUTION SYSTEM

Pressure in the Arteries

The aorta and arteries offer little resistance to flow of blood, consequently, the gradient of pressure along them is small. The arterial system is subject to hydrostatic changes; therefore when a man stands up the arterial pressure in his feet is increased by the hydrostatic pressure difference between his feet and his heart. This pressure is about 130 cm. H_2O (95 mm. Hg); so the pressure in his dorsalis pedis artery would arise from 120/80 to 215/175. The effect of this rise of pressure is offset by an equal rise in venous pressure; nevertheless blood flow to the feet is favored by the upright posture. The effect of gravitational factors on arterial pressure in terms of blood flow is seen even more clearly when the arm is elevated above heart level. In this

3

case the venous pressure, being near atmospheric pressure, cannot be greatly reduced, and the effects of local reduction of arterial pressure on the blood flow to the tissues are more clearly seen. Blood flow falls with the reduction in arterial pressure, and there is no evidence of compensatory dilatation of the resistance vessels. If the muscles of the elevated limb are exercised an accumulation of metabolites results in local dilatation, but the resultant hyperemia is restricted, and pain or fatigue occurs in the exercising muscles.

The hydrostatic effect is important to remember in the nursing of an ischemic limb. Although elevation may reduce the edema, it will result in an intensification of the ischemia, whereas dependency will diminish the ischemia if adequate venous drainage can be ensured. This principle should be impressed on all who are concerned in the nursing of patients with peripheral vascular disease.

Arterial Flow Through an Obstruction

The most prevalent arterial disease, atheroma, produces resistance to arterial flow by narrowing major arteries. The physical relations affecting flow through a narrowed section of a tube have been described in terms of Poiseuille's equation:

$$\text{Flow} = \frac{K \text{ (pressure gradient over constriction) (radius of constriction)}^4}{\text{(length of the constriction) (viscosity of blood)}}$$

This equation was derived from empirical data on laminar flow of fluid through rigid tubes of fixed caliber. Its value in relation to arterial obstruction is that it calls attention to the factors which should be considered. Our own attempts to apply it to flow through an arterial constriction foundered on our inability to measure in situ the internal diameter of a constricted vessel with the exactitude required if such a small measurement is to be raised to the fourth power.

The other factor which is difficult to measure is the viscosity of blood. Blood viscosity is affected by its hematocrit, the internal viscosity of the red cell, the degree of red cell aggregation, plasma viscosity, and flow velocity. At low flow velocities blood may be 1,000 times more viscous than water, but at high velocities only 2 to 4 times more viscous. This remarkable property is related to the extremely low internal viscosity of the red cells, which becomes more evident as red cell aggregates formed at low velocity flows disperse when the flow rate is increased. Thus blood has a high viscosity when flowing slowly through the veins and a low viscosity when moving at a faster rate through arteries. It may be expected to have an even lower viscosity in the rapid flow through an arterial obstruction. This last supposition may contribute to the surprising experimental finding that a segmental obstruction may encroach on three fourths of the arterial lumen before a pressure gradient and reduction of flow occurs.

Another phenomenon which must be taken into account in consideration of flow through a stenosis is that of turbulent flow. Turbulence is encouraged by the irregularities of the arterial intima caused by atheroma and more by the increase in flow velocity of the blood through a stenosis. The change from an orderly laminar flow to a disorderly turbulent one is associated with a marked increase in resistance to flow. Often the associated vibrations reach audible intensity and give rise to a systolic bruit over the stenosis. Turbulent flow had been eliminated in the design of Poiseuille's experiments and is not considered in the formula, but it cannot be eliminated in diseased arteries. It was studied by Reynolds a century ago. He found that velocity is of first importance, but also to be taken into account are the viscosity and density of the fluid, and the radius of the tube through which it is flowing. These factors are combined in the Reynolds Number, which is an index without dimensions. When conditions are such that this number is exceeded, turbulent flow is likely to supervene.

The factor of turbulence was taken into account in an informative series of observations carried out by Schultz et al. They investigated pressure-flow relationships in normal and atherosclerotic aortoiliac segments removed at autopsy. They used a pulsatile perfusion system in order to simulate conditions in the living body. In normal vessels only small pressure gradients were set up as the flow velocity was increased. The pressure-volume flow relationship appeared to be linear and of the magnitude to be expected in a system in which laminar flow was occurring. In the atherosclerotic arteries different results were obtained. As the flow rate was increased over the same range a point was reached at which the pressure gradient began to increase sharply. For example, in one specimen with a reduction of only 6 per cent of cross sectional area there was a 12 mm. Hg pressure gradient when the volume of flow had been increased to 40 ml./sec. To explain why the vascular resistance had become so much greater than it had been in the normal specimen, it is suggested that at this rate of blood flow the stream had become turbulent and that turbulence would increase with increasing flow rates. Thus, the decreased viscosity of the blood which results from the faster flow rate through an obstruction is countered by the increased resistance to flow caused by the development of turbulence. These are important observations when considering diseased vessels in man.

Collateral Circulation

Within recent years the normal functioning of the collateral circulation has been newly appreciated. Its functioning is most strikingly shown in the maintenance of constant blood flow to the cerebral circulation. This blood flow is maintained by the system of anastomoses between carotid and vertebral arteries known as the circle of Willis. As the head turns and bends on the neck, and the neck on the shoulders, one or another of the carotid or vertebral arteries is liable to be obstructed, but the blood supply to the brain is not diminished because of the ease by which blood can flow by an alternate route. Whether the flow goes directly or round by the collateral circulation depends on the pressure gradient within the arteries. When the main vessel is sufficiently occluded there is a fall of distal pressure with a resultant increase in pressure gradient over the collateral vessels and an increased flow through them.

With permanent arterial block, as with atheroma, blood flows as directed by the pressure gradient. The best known example is when there is an obstruction of the first part of the subclavian artery with a fall of pressure in the artery distally. Since the left vertebral artery takes origin in the second part of the subclavian artery, the pressure here is reduced compared to that in the basilar artery to which the right vertebral artery also flows. Consequently, blood flows up the right vertebral to the basilar and down the left vertebral into the left subclavian and axillary artery. This example of reversal of flow direction through the left vertebral artery was named subclavian steal by an astute editor; the name is a good one for the anastomoses normally required to protect the supply of blood to the brain are in these cases taking blood away from the brain.

The collateral systems in the circulation to the limbs do not offer so generous an alternate blood supply as do those to the brain, presumably because the tissues of the limbs are able to withstand longer periods of relative ischemia than the brain. In locations where the main artery may be compressed by acute flexion of a joint or by pressure from moving ligamentous or bony structures, alternative pathways exist. Examples are the arterial anastomoses around the knee and elbow joints which provide for distal flow should the main artery become kinked by acute flexion of the joint.

When permanent block of the main artery results in prolonged increase of flow through the collateral vessels, the latter dilate and hypertrophy. The increase in caliber of the collateral circulation takes place slowly. Ludbrook investigated the vascular resistance of collateral circulation in patients with intermittent claudication. Collateral circulation produced 23 per cent of the total resistance at rest and 73 per cent with peak flows. Moreover, if the peripheral resistance of the terminal arterioles was abolished, the maximum blood flow increased only about 10 per cent. The relative importance of factors which lead to the facilitation of flow through the collateral vessels is still undetermined. To be considered are the accumulation of metabolites with vasodilator properties in the ischemic tissues, a continuing increased pressure gradient along the collateral vessel, and the possible effects of neural influences.

Reactivity of Arteries

When a muscular artery is subjected to trauma, whether it be physical, such as a puncture or involvement in bone fracture or chemical such as an injection of thiopental into it, there is a real danger that it will go into spasm. Such occurrences are dramatic, and fortunately uncommon, but they greatly influenced conceptions of arterial disease at one time, and "arterial spasm" was held to be responsible for intermittent claudication, blanching of the skin of an ischemic limb, or transient attacks of cerebral ischemia. Other, more convincing explanations have been given for these phenomena and the concept of arterial spasm became less popular except in the obvious and dramatic response to trauma.

RESISTANCE SYSTEM: ARTERIOLES

Organs such as the heart and brain require a constant and adequate blood supply; other organs such as the gastrointestinal tract and skeletal muscles need increased flow only during activity and a much less or even intermittent flow during resting periods. Circulation is maintained to organs which need a constant supply and otherwise directed to organs in most need of it by means of a regulatory system. In this system the means by which flow is directed to or away from tissues lies in the resistance vessels or arterioles. The patency of the arterioles is affected by nervous, humoral or physical stimuli, and arterioles of different tissues respond to different degrees to these various influences. For example, increase of blood flow to active muscle is by means of vasoactive metabolites produced within the muscle, but when muscles are resting the blood flow through them is largely controlled by nervous and hormonal stimuli. The arterioles and arteriovenous anastomoses of the digital circulation are largely controlled by nervous impulses but they are affected also by circulating vasoactive substances and by the physical stimuli of heat and cold. It may be that the blood vessels of erectile genital tissue are controlled entirely by nervous stimuli. In general terms it is almost true to say that when the circulatory needs of the body as a whole are to be met, nervous impulses control the changes while vasoactive substances locally produced are responsible for local increases in blood flow.

In the following paragraphs we are concerned with the control of blood flow through the arterioles of the limbs. For practical purposes this means the arterioles of the skin and the muscles, for little is known of the regulation of blood flow through skeletal and connective tissue.

Regulation of Blood Flow Through Skin

There is a general lack of appreciation amongst clinicians of the difference of the circulatory reactions of the skin covering the digits and that covering the arm, forearm, thigh, and calf. The circulation in the digits is directed to the requirement of the body for losing or conserving heat. The system is a highly specialized organ and is remarkably sensitive to all forms of stimuli. Further to emphasize the uniqueness of this difference I have placed the discussion of the structure and function of this thermoregulatory organ in Chapter 8, where the unique properties of the digital circulation are considered in relation to digital ischemia.

The phenomenon of the axone reflex, however, is shared by both digital and proximal skin; this is the flare response to injury. Arterioles in the skin are innervated by branches of the sensory afferent fibers, probably "C" pain fibers. Stimuli which damage the skin, such as needle prick, a burn, or contact with a noxious chemical, produce the sensation of pain and also a dilatation of the nearby arterioles. This response depends on the integrity of the peripheral nerves and is due to an axone reflex. Its value in the protection of the integument is undoubted; when it is lost, as in diabetic neuropathy, the skin is particularly liable to damage from noxious stimuli.

In comparison with the highly reactive digital circulation that of the proximal skin is nonreactive. Observations of the reactivity of its arterioles to such stimuli as body heating, or blocking of peripheral or sympathetic pathways have always been interpreted in the implicit belief that skin much have a vasomotor supply from the autonomic nervous system. It is instructive to reconsider these results with a more open mind.

In man body heating sufficient to cause a small increase in temperature of blood flowing through the midbrain stimulates autonomic reflexes to increase the loss of heat from the body. The responses are an increase of blood flow in the skin of the hands and feet and thermal sweating. The former is initiated by even mild body heating, the latter requires more intense body heating. Sympathetic denervation of the limbs removes the efferent path of both these reflexes.

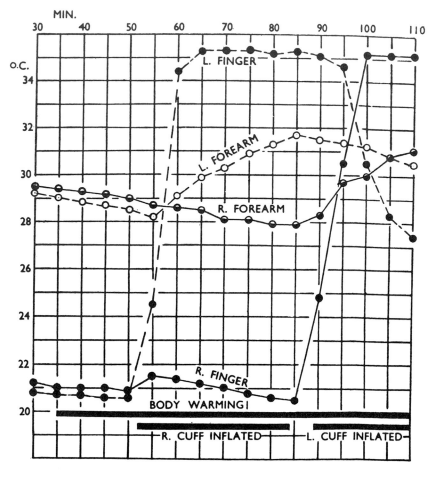

The increase in peripheral skin flow could be caused by relaxation of vasoconstrictor tone or stimulation of vasodilator fibers. Evidence points only to the former and indicates that this change takes place only in the circulation of the hands and feet and in the superficial veins draining those extremities. If release of neural vasoconstriction of the more proximal skin of the arms and legs occurs, the evidence for it is uncertain. We were unable to show any such effect (Fig. 1-1). Further we were unable to demonstrate any increase in skin temperature on blocking the mixed cutaneous nerves to the forearm or calf. In these experiments the precaution was taken of preventing the return circulation of warm blood from the hands and feet by inflating wrist or ankle cuffs.

On the other hand, Roddie et al. observed a small increase in forearm blood flow on body heating even before the occurrence of sweating, suggesting neural activity either by vasodilator fibers or by release of vasoconstrictor tone. There were, however, two important differences in technique. In Roddie's experiments the circulation to and from the hand appears to have been unrestricted except during the actual measurement of blood flow.

Fig. 1-1. Effect of body heating on skin temperature of forearm. As body heating commenced pneumatic cuffs were placed on both wrists. (*Left*) The skin temperature of the left fingers and forearm rose normally. At the 90th minute, the cuff on the left wrist was inflated so that warm blood from the hand no longer passed through the cutaneous veins of the forearm. The skin temperature of the forearm began to fall, though body heating continued. (*Right*) On the right side venous return from the hand had been prevented by inflation of the wrist cuff, and there had been no rise in skin temperature of fingers or forearm, When the cuff on the right wrist was released at 90 minutes, the hand warmed up promptly, and a secondary rise in skin temperature occurred in the forearm skins. These observations, and others similar, led to the idea that unless body heating is severe enough to provoke sweating no direct warming occurs in the skin of the proximal portions of the limbs but only a secondary warming because of the return of warm venous blood from the hands. (From Grant, R. T. and Pearson, R. S. B.: Clin. Sci., *3*:119, 1938.)

Under these circumstances the opening up of A-V anastomoses in the hands results in an inflow of warm arterial blood into the plexus of superficial forearm veins so that the skin is warmed in a secondary manner and the cutaneous vessels relax. The other difference is that the degree of heating used by Roddie was sufficient to promote sudomotor activity, and marked dilatation of the arterioles of the forearm skin occurs when body heating is sufficiently intense to cause sweating. Blocking the cutaneous nerves to the forearm or calf prevents this dilatation if done before body heating, and reverses it if done during body heating.

Our original interpretation of these results was that the increase in blood flow was due to the stimulation of vasodilator nerves. Subsequently, Fox and Hilton provided evidence for the more plausible explanation that the increase in blood flow is due to the vasodilator effect of bradykinin which diffuses from active sweat glands. Their observations are also consistent with the occurrence of an increase in skin blood flow from this cause before the appearance of sweating, for with this intense heating they observed an increase in the bradykinin content of perfusate from the subcutaneous space and an increase in skin temperature before the outbreak of demonstrable sweating.

In summary, investigations of possible vasomotor activity in the skin of the forearm and calf do not clearly demonstrate any primary activity of vasomotor nerves, so the existence of vasomotor supply to the skin remains questionable. The subject has its practical application in assessing the benefit to be expected from sympathectomy and will be further considered under that heading.

Regulation of Blood Flow Through Muscle

In general terms the blood flow through resting muscle is controlled by physical, neurogenic, and hormonal influences; all of which appear to be subservient to the requirements of the general circulation rather than the needs of muscle tissue. The hyperemia of actively contracting muscle, even though it results from an extremely potent vasodilator metabolite, can still be modified by the physical, neurogenic and hormonal factors.

There is evidence that one path of the bloodstream through muscle tissue passes through the microcirculation and subserves its nutritional requirements; another pathway bypasses the microcirculation and appears to act as a buffer system for the general circulation. Histological evidence for the two circulations is lacking, but if the flow through the arcades of small vessels in an exposed muscle is observed through a microscope it is not difficult to believe that pathways exist by means of which portions of the bloodstream can bypass the microcirculation. Functional evidence for the two circulations depends on discrepancies between measured blood flow and either the rate of clearance of Na^{24} from the tissues or the uptake of oxygen by the muscle. Epinephrine, for example, causes an increase in blood flow through muscle which has little or no effect on either the uptake of oxygen or of Na^{24}, and hyperthyroidism results in an increase of blood flow to muscle far greater than required for any increase of metabolism of the muscle.

The temperature of muscle has a strong effect on the blood flow through it. A cold muscle has little flow, a warm muscle more than enough to supply its metabolic requirements (Table 1-1). The increase in blood flow with increased muscle temperature is a factor which contributes to increase muscle flow during muscular exercise, for contraction is an exothermic process and results in an increase in the local muscle temperature.

The resistance vessels of muscle act as a buffer to the circulation in that they accommodate arterial thrusts of pressure and volume. This is seen when the left ventricular output suddenly becomes excessive as when a large A-V fistula is suddenly closed or when tourniquets are suddenly applied to three limbs. In the case of the A-V fistula closure, a brief increase in forearm and calf blood

TABLE 1-1. LOCAL MUSCLE TEMPERATURE AND
FOREARM BLOOD FLOW

Temperature (°C.)	15	20	25	30	35	43
Blood Flow (ml./100 ml./min.)	0.5	0.6	0.9	1.9	3.5	16.0

flow occurs immediately; in the case of the tourniquets on the three limbs, a brief increase in flow takes place in the muscles of the remaining limb.

Muscle tissue also accommodates to reduced arterial pressure and blood flow. We lowered the perfusion pressure in the forearm by elevating the limb and found a linear relationship between brachial blood pressure and forearm blood flow. Burton and Yamada found a similar relationship when the effective brachial arterial pressure was reduced by increasing the pressure within the plethysmograph to increase tissue pressure. In these experiments no indication of vasodilatation in the forearm vessels was observed to compensate for the reduction in arterial pressure, and the oxygen uptake of the muscles was maintained by an increase in the coefficient of oxygen utilization. No reactive hyperemia followed the period of reduced flow. It appears that the alteration in level of blood flow under these circumstances is a passive physical result of the reduction of perfusion pressure.

Observations of the effects of chronic reduction of perfusion pressure presents obvious difficulties. In patients with intermittent claudication with predominantly unilateral vascular disease we have observed wasting of the muscles of the affected limb. The wasting appears to progress until the reduced volume of muscle is comparable to the reduced volume of resting blood flow, for the level of this measurement (ml./100 ml./min.) is found to be similar in the two limbs. In judging the value of this observation one must take into account the relative disuse of the muscles of the affected limb.

The effect of diminished perfusion pressure on the hyperemia of exercise is shown by plethysmographic measurements (Fig. 1-2). Resting flow may be within normal limits, but the increase in blood flow following exercise is slight and is slow to reach its low maximum. It is clear that full dilatation of the resistance vessels is unable to compensate for the arterial obstruction.

Neurogenic Influences. Evidence that the blood vessels of human muscles are innervated by sympathetic nerve fibers was shown by the twofold increase in blood flow which occurred in forearm muscles when the mixed nerves to them had been

BLOOD FLOW BEFORE AND AFTER EXERCISE.

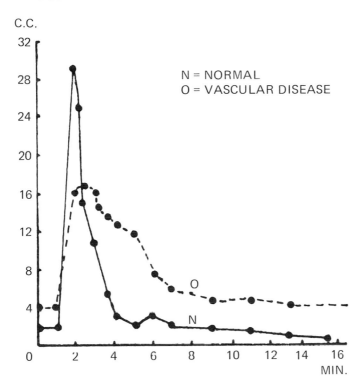

Fig. 1-2. Hyperemia of exercise. After one minute's exercise of the muscles of the normal forearm a prompt and intense hyperemia occurs which has subsided 3 minutes after cessation of the exercise. After the same amount of exercise of the muscles of the other arm with block of the brachial artery the hyperemia is delayed, reaches only half the intensity, and persists for twice as long. (From Grant, R. T.: Clin. Sci., 3:157, 1938.)

blocked by anesthesia. The increase did not occur in sympathectomised limbs (Barcroft and Edholm 1943).

One of the functions of this innervation is to maintain arterial pressure during postural changes. Tilting a normal person from the horizontal to the vertical position is accompanied by vasoconstriction in the forearm vessels. Raising the lower trunk and legs of a recumbent subject results in an increase in forearm blood flow. These reactions are presumed due to sympathetic impulses, since they could not be demonstrated after such denervation. The reflex is absent also in idiopathic orthostatic hypotension. A contrary reaction is seen during fainting (vaso-vagal syncope) when an increase in forearm blood flow occurs. In these circumstances the blood flow in a normally innervated arm is greater than that in one in which radial, ulnar, and median nerves have been blocked. For this reason the action of sympathetic vasodilator nerves rather than the simple release of vasoconstrictor tone is suggested. The afferent stimuli for these reflexes appear to arise from baroceptors in the right and left atria, and probably also in the pulmonary circulation.

Vasodilatation in the vessels of limb muscles during emotional stress has been said to be mediated by sympathetic cholinergic fibers and by a humoral agent, possibly epinephrine. From a parallel series of experiments and from a reconsideration of the data of the previous workers I deduced that the vasodilatation was not directly mediated by nervous impulses. Cholinergic vasodilatation (probably through the activity of sweat glands) may occasionally occur, but the usual response appears to be due to a humoral agent which is unlikely to be epinephrine.

Humoral Agents. Epinephrine has been the most closely studied of humoral agents which affect the resistance vessels of muscle. The response is a complicated one. When dilute epinephrine is infused intravenously, tachycardia, a slight decrease in arterial pressure, and a large increase in forearm blood flow occurs. This happens after a delay of about a minute and is transient. An increase in pulse pressure follows with a lessening of the increase in pulse rate and blood flow to the forearm. When epinephrine in very dilute solution is infused intraarterially the blood flow after the transient increase is often less than in the control period. The effects seen with epinephrine appear to be due to a mixture of vasodilator and vasoconstrictor effects of the amine further complicated by different responses to different dose levels. The brief latent period before a response occurs has not been satisfactorily explained.

Norepinephrine constricts muscle vessels.

The effect of many other agents in blood flow of muscle have been observed and it is relevant to remark that none compare in potency with the vasodilator effects of the metabolites of muscular contraction. The more active ones: epinephrine, adenosine triphosphate, histamine, and acetylcholine may double the rate of blood flow through resting muscle but are still without effect on the amount and rate of blood flow-debt repayment following rhythmic exercise of the muscles. Translated into clinical practice this means that vasodilator agents now known are a drop in the ocean compared to the vasodilator action of exercise.

Sympathectomy

The hyperemic effects of sympathectomy were recorded over a century ago by Claude Bernard. The following is a free translation from his "Leçons des Liquides de L'Organism" pp. 250-251 (1859). "I have severed the main sympathetic trunk in the neck of a guinea pig. . . . when the ear on that side is seen in transmitted light it is found to be very much more vascular than on the normal side, and this occurs in rabbits and other animals. . . . After sympathetic section temperature rises in the area and [venous] blood remains red. If the sympathetic trunk is stimulated the. . . . part cools and venous blood becomes very dark." The striking effect which Bernard described is due to removal of sympathetic vasoconstrictor tone from specialized organs (A-V anastomoses). These organs in the rabbit's ear are concerned with regulation of body temperature, and their anatomical structure was not described until three years later (Sucquet, see Chap. 8). Of particular interest, therefore, is that Bernard mentions arterialization of venous blood as if the possibility of A-V connections was in his mind.

In the century succeeding Bernard's observations a difference of opinion has arisen concerning the effects of sympathetic neurectomy. The physiologist who has made measurements of blood flow day by day immediately after sympathectomy is encouraged to take the position: "Loss of vessel tone after sympathetic denervation is only temporary; within about two weeks the tone is only slightly less than the preoperative value so that the greatly increased flow after surgery rapidly subsides to nearly the preoperative level" (Dr. John Shepherd 1963). On the other hand, a surgeon who has seen ischemic toes begin to heal after a lumbar sympathectomy is encouraged to consider the operation as "the most certain means of producing long lasting vasodilatation that we possess." This quotation is from Sir Thomas Lewis in 1936, though I doubt whether he would have made such a statement in 1946, and almost certainly not in 1956 when more certain means of increasing blood flow to a limb had become available.

An explanation for these two differing opinions of the effect of sympathectomy may be given by considering the immediate postoperative effect of sympathectomy on the blood flow to the proximal and distal parts of a limb and the long term effect on the distal parts.

In 1938 we reported skin temperatures and blood flows in limbs in the days immediately after sympathectomy, and separated the effects in proximal parts from those in more distal. The operated limb was dry and hot after operation but by the third day the hyperemia of the proximal skin had begun to subside and was gone by the 18th day. The hand in one case and the foot in another remained warmer than on the unoperated side even though the intense hyperemia which had been observed shortly after operation had largely subsided. Subsequently Barcroft confirmed and amplified these findings, and Dornhorst and Sharpey-Schafer measured the effects of sympathectomy on the collateral circulation in a limb. These careful observers all agreed that the blood flow through proximal tissues of a limb, be it skin, muscle, or collateral circulation is increased two- to threefold after sympathetic neurectomy, but that the hyperemia falls to control levels after two weeks. In the hands and feet the sequence of events is similar except that the immediate hyperemia is more intense and some degree of hyperemia persists. Of particular interest is that the maximum hyperemia in hand and foot is not seen immediately but is delayed for 24 to 48 hours, the delay being longer in the feet than in the hands.

Various theories have been advanced to explain the subsidence of the hyperemia in the first two weeks after sympathectomy. These have mostly been concerned with mechanisms for the return of vessel tone. An alternate theory derives from the suggestion of Trotter and Davies that the hyperesthesia following nerve section is accounted for by liberation of irritative substances from degenerating nerves. Following this idea, sympathetic section may have a dilator effect other than by the simple removal of constrictor influences. The delay observed in attainment of maximum hyperemia in hand and foot suggests that some process consequent upon nerve section but not its immediate effect is the cause of the early hyperemia. In the skin of the forearm and calf we see hyperemia after sympathectomy even though we have otherwise found no evidence for vasoconstrictor tone in these areas. For these reasons the hypothesis that the intense and overall hyperemia following sympathectomy is due to release of vasodilator substances subsequent to degeneration of sympathetic nerves and end organs is worthy of further investigation. So far this hypothesis has no direct experimental support.

It remains to explain why vasodilatation in hands and feet after sympathectomy is more permanent. In these regions there is very active vasoconstrictor control of the A-V anastomoses. In the rabbit's ear these have been seen to open up after sympathetic nerve section, and it is presumably the ablation of vasoconstrictor tone from them in the digits which accounts for the longer lasting hyperemia of the extremities. Even this hyperemia abates, however, for particularly in the hand and to a lesser degree in the foot connections between the central sympathetic supply and the periphery are slowly reestablished.

This brief account of the complex phenomena which have been observed to follow sympathetic neurectomy will have served a purpose if it emphasizes that the increased blood flow to a limb which follows the operations lasts only about 2 weeks and only in the hands and feet is a longer lasting hyperemia achieved.

MICROCIRCULATION

Anatomy and Physiology

As the named arteries branch into smaller arteries the lumina of the branches eventually narrow to a cross section so small that the vessel may be termed an arteriole. The distinction is one not only of size but of function, for the arteriole is the prime resistance vessel and as such is extremely responsive to stimuli: neural, hormonal, or physical. Just at what diameter an artery becomes an arteriole is an arbitrary distinction, for the transition is a gradual one. The smaller arteries interconnect in a series of arcades. As this system merges into the microcirculation the interconnections become even more numerous so that the microcirculation presents as a network, albeit in three dimensions. Different vessels have been distinguished as arising from the interbranching of arterioles:

1. Metarterioles—microscopic vessels which have a sparse and discontinuous muscular coat.

2. Capillaries—endothelial tubes with a muscular sphincter only at their origin from the arteriole.

3. A-V anastomoses—short thick-walled channels with a well formed muscular coat.

4. Thoroughfare or preferential channels of similar dimensions to capillaries but with a continuous muscular coat over half their length.

Recent studies of the microcirculation have stressed that the venous or capacitance side is 20 times larger in volume and cross sectional area than the arterial or resistance side. In consequence of this larger cross sectional area, flow through the venules slows, and the viscous resistance to flow is very high. Aggregations of red cells are very liable to occur here which further increase resistance to flow. In the opinion of some workers the route and rate of flow through the microcirculation is controlled more by changes in the venous than in the arterial side.

Nerve fibers can be seen in close association with the vessels of the microcirculation. In human skin the branches of somatic afferent fibers innervate the arterioles; the action of this innervation is seen in the "triple response." Sympathetic vasoconstrictor control exists over the A-V anastomoses of the skin of the hands, feet and face, but these are specialized organs concerned with thermal regulation. Sympathetic vasoconstrictor impulses also control the resistance vessels of the arterioles of voluntary muscle. To what degree nervous impulses control other vessels of the microcirculation is not known; perhaps precapillary sphincters are innervated, or perhaps changes in them are secondary to those at the arteriolar level. Judging by the responses of a denervated circulation, most of the functions can be activated by physical and chemical influences.

The naming of the vessels becomes irrelevant as one sees the microcirculation in function in any tissue which can be transilluminated. The impression through the microscope is of a constantly changing pattern of activity. Cellular elements of the blood are seen to change their shape as they are squeezed through narrow channels. In other channels the axial stream of corpuscles flows, whereas in still others masses of cells pile up in temporary stasis. Distinction between metarterioles and venules may be difficult to make out, for the structure of the wall cannot be clearly seen and changes of pressure gradient at the ends of the vessels result in reversal of the direction of flow in some vessels.

The traffic pattern seen indicates a continually changing relationship between filtration and reabsorption in individual vessels of the microcirculation. The blood which flows through the A-V anastomoses or preferential channels will have no opportunity for exchange of solutes with the tissues. A steady stream of corpuscles flowing through a capillary implies a high intraluminal pressure that exceeds the sum of tissue and colloid osmotic pressure resulting in filtration of solutes from the blood. When the precapillary sphincter contracts pressure within, the capillary falls and flow through it slows so that physical conditions favor the reabsorption of tissue fluid and solutes.

Four possible mechanisms of transcapillary exchange of solutes and particles with the tissues have been described: (1) physical filtration occurring through pores in the intercellular element of the capillary wall; (2) some exchange of solutes may take place directly through the endothelial cells of the capillary wall; (3) exchange of material by "pinocytosis," that is, engulfing of particles by microvacuoles at one endothelial surface and movement of the vacuole through the cell to discharge its load through the opposite wall; (4) phagocytosis of colloid particles by macrophages on one side of the endothelium and a break through the cell barrier and discharge of the particles on the other side of it. All these mechanisms of transfer seem to be very slow, but the large area of the interface between blood and tissues presented by the capillaries must make the process adequate for metabolic requirements.

Microcirculation in Man in Health and Disease

The microcirculation can be observed in the conjunctivae, mucosa, and nail folds. Most attention has been directed to the venous effluent of the capillary loops which are more visible and show greater changes in disease states. Sir Thomas Lewis was an early observer of the microcirculation in the skin. He investigated the vascular reaction of the "triple response" as reaction to minor injury. This consists of a central red spot or streak, due to capillary dilatation; transudation of fluid with formation of a wheal or blister; and a surrounding bright red flare with ill-defined margins attributable to the arteriolar dilatation of an axone reflex.

Most investigations of the microcirculation have described morphological changes which can be observed without experimental intervention. Dilatation of the venous side of the capillary loop has been described with aging and to be more pronounced when the patient has diabetes, hyperlipidemia, coronary artery disease, or cerebrovascular disease. Changes are also seen in "collagen vascular disease." A correlation has been shown between the degree of abnormality in the conjunctival microcirculation and the severity of coronary arterial disease in respect to both flow and morphology. Similarly with cerebrovascular disease. Many patients with primary types III and IV hyperlipoproteinemia show significantly more dilated venous loops than control subjects. Electron microscopy of microcirculation in tissues removed from diabetic patients has shown thickening of the basement membrane, but the relationship of this to dilatation of the venous capillary loop is not clear.

Extension of these investigations may be hoped for. Observations could be made on the effects of changes of experimental conditions on the abnormalities seen. Histological studies using injection digestion techniques may be expected to demonstrate pathological changes in excised tissues, and electron microscopy to show the more intimate details of alterations in vessel walls. Measurement of dysfunction may then be related to changes in structure.

COLLECTING AND CAPACITANCE

Microcirculation to Veins

From the venous loops of the microcirculation blood passes into a venous plexus of collecting channels. The details of this plexus cannot be seen by the naked eye, but, in the absence of natural or applied skin pigmentation, it is the amount and color of the blood in the plexus which gives color to human skin. Animal preparations—bat's wing, rabbit ear chamber, hamster cheek pouch, etc.—have been used for the purpose of studying pressure and flow in this plexus. It has been observed that an increased resistance to flow can occur which is independent of changes at the arteriolar level. If the resistance to flow in these microscopic veins is increased, pressure rises in the capillaries, flow through them slows, and there is an increase in transudation of fluid.

The first order of veins arises from this plexus. Under the skin they can be seen to form a reticular pattern, especially when seen by infrared photography. From this network the collecting veins arise. On the hands and forearms particularly, and on the feet and calves to a lesser degree, the subcutaneous veins form an elaborate network which is concerned with regulation of body heat. From the network of veins in the muscles the deep venous channels arise. The superficial and deep veins are connected by frequent communicating veins.

Capacitance Function

The named veins of the limbs, the veins of the organs, and the venae cavae provide the venous capacitance system. The functioning of this depends on changes in compliance of the venous wall which is the ease with which it will stretch when the pressure within it increases. The compliance of the veins is in part dependent on their intrinsic elastic properties, but it is also greatly influenced by the tone of the smooth muscle within the wall. Innervations of this muscle is by alpha (constrictor) receptors. No evidence for beta (dilator) receptors has been produced. Increase of tone of the smooth muscle affects the cross sectional area of the vein, the capacity of the venous reservoir, and the rate of blood flow through it. Study of the capacity function of the great veins is more logically concerned with cardiac function, but insofar as it affects the velocity of flow through the major veins it can be considered here.

The assessment of venous tone depends on the measurement of the relation between pressure and volume increments in the veins. One method used is to empty the veins of a limb by the application of external pressure. The limb, or rather a portion of the limb, is surrounded by a rigid plethysmograph. The water pressure in the plethysmograph is raised to 15 mm. Hg, which results in an initial effective venous pressure of 1 mm. Hg and a reduction of venous volume from 3.0 to 0.6 ml./100 ml. of forearm. Increases of pressure to 30 or 40 mm. Hg express but little more blood from the limb. The veins are then congested by the application of a standard series of pressure increments in a congesting cuff proximal to the plethysmograph. The increase in venous volume at each step is measured by the increase in limb volume and the pressure within the veins by that in the congesting cuff. By this means the pressure-volume relationship can be observed under different conditions. The method appears to be simple but requires close attention to detail.

Venous Valves

In the history of the circulation the importance of the venous valves in preventing retrograde venous flow was an important point in the development of Harvey's concept of the circulation. The proper function of the venous valves is as important to the onward flow of blood against gravity as is the functioning of heart valves in the passage of blood through the heart. In the case of the veins the force required to impel blood along them is provided by the contractions of the limb muscles surrounding them. It is the deep system which is active in venous return against gravity, for the muscle pump is much less effective in the case of the superficial veins; however, valves in the communicating veins are arranged so that blood can pass from the superficial to deep veins as the latter are emptied and more effective use is made of the muscle pump. The effectiveness of this pump is seen in measurements of venous pressure at the ankle. When a man stands still the venous pressure at the ankles rises to some 100 mm. Hg, but as the pumping action of the calf muscles comes into play blood in the deep veins is impelled towards the heart and replaced by blood flowing from the distended superficial veins. In this manner the pressure in the superficial veins at the ankle falls from 100 mm. Hg to 30 mm. Hg during the action of the muscles, only to rise again if the action ceases.

When venous valves of the deep system have become incompetent as a result of venous thrombosis the effectiveness of the muscle pump is greatly reduced. When the patient sits or stands for a long time blood drains into the veins of the feet and lower calves, and the pressure within them rises creating a secondary rise in capillary pressure and increased transudation of fluid occurs with the formation of edema. With normal deep venous valves minor contractions of the muscles of the calves diminish the full effect of the increased pressure, but when the valves are incompetent, this relief is not available and edema fluid forms at an increased rate. In the treatment of patients with incompetent valves of the leg veins, it is customary to use some form of elastic support stocking. The firm external support of the stocking makes the muscle pump more effective on the subcutaneous veins, the distention of the veins is limited so blood flows at a greater velocity along them, and by limiting the expansion of the leg the formation of edema is limited. The elastic support cannot fully compensate for the incompetence of the valves, but it greatly reduces its consequences.

LYMPHATIC SYSTEM

Between 1620 and 1630 two outstanding discoveries in the study of circulation occurred. William Harvey's observations of the circulation led him to the knowledge that blood circulates from arteries to veins and through the heart, and Gasparo Aselli first described the circulation of the lymph.

While the understanding of blood circulation advanced slowly in the succeeding years virtually nothing new was learned about the lymphatic circulation. Accounts of its anatomy appear in 1787 (Mascagni) and again in 1874 (Sappey), but interest in the functions of the lymphatic system did not become aroused until Drinker, stimulated by Starling's work, began experimental studies in animals. In the last 15 years study of the function of the lymphatics has generated intense interest. Much of this interest has been directed to the role of the lymphatic system in countering invasion of the body by foreign materials, but there has also been great interest in the study of mechanisms of lymph formation and disposal. The formation of lymph, that is, the passage of protein-rich fluid from the capillary lumen to tissue spaces is recognized as providing transport for substances such as iron, lipoproteins and antibodies, and is no less essential to the healthy body than the passage of oxygen from red cells to tissues.

The lymphatic system may be regarded as an offshoot of the collecting venous system with the function of returning to the circulation from the tissue fluid nearly all the protein and other macromolecules which cannot be directly reabsorbed into blood capillaries. Like the venous system the lymphatic system has valves and depends on the muscle pump for movement of lymph against the force of gravity.

The lymphatics originate as a fine network of small collecting capillaries in all tissues with a well developed blood supply. In spite of microscopic observations of lymphatics in such preparations as the rabbit's or mouse's ear, and electron microscopy of the tissues there is still doubt concerning the means by which macromolecules and even colloids pass from tissue fluids into the lymphatics. Molecules of weight greater than 2,000 cannot leak from the lymphatics, but smaller molecules can as can be seen by the red streak of lymphangitis or the white streak which outlines the lymphatic path when epinephrine has been injected subcutaneously. These appearances are due to vasodilatation in the first case and vasoconstriction in the second of the vasa vasorum of the adventitial layers of the lymphatics caused by the leakage of the vasoactive substances.

The peripheral lymphatics join into larger lymphatics and pass through regional lymph nodes before reaching the bloodstream. Because of the high permeability of the lymphatic pathways the lymph undergoes progressive concentration as it flows on to join the bloodstream. Afferent lymphatics enter the node by an oblique course through the cortex, and the efferent lymphatic (for it usually is single) leaves by the medulla or pelvis. The afferent lymphatics are considerably larger in diameter than the efferent vessel as the volume of inflow of lymph into the node is significantly higher than the outflow. "The regional lymph node is an organ redistributing fluid between the venous and lymphatic systems in accord with the anatomical and functional state of the lymphatic and venous channels" (Borodin and Tomchik). Within the node particles such as carbon (India ink or coal dust), microorganisms, or neoplastic cells are filtered out of the lymph before it returns to the main blood stream.

The usual teaching is that the return of lymph into the main stream occurs where the thoracic duct opens into the venous system near the left subclavian-jugular junction. The anatomy of the lymphatic system, however, is quite variable and communications between lymphatic and venous systems exist in other regions of the body. In the thoracic and abdominal regions many lymphatico-venous communications exist at which regurgitation of blood into the lymphatic is prevented by long leafed semilunar bicuspid valves. Flow of lymph into the veins at these junctions is intermittent and may be stimulated by pharmacological or neural stimuli.

The wide variations that have been reported in rates of lymph formation flow and pressures may be attributed to the many factors which affect measurement and interpretation of the readings. Spontaneous rhythmic contractions of larger lymphatics have been demonstrated during cine-lymphangiography, but the genesis of these contractions and their effectiveness in propulsion of the lymph flow remains in doubt.

REFERENCES

General

Strandness, D.E., Jr. ed.: Collateral Circulation in Clinical Surgery. Philadelphia, W. B. Saunders, 1969.

Viscosity of Whole Blood

Dintenfass, L.: Blood Microrheology. New York, Appleton-Century Crofts, 1971.

Flow Through a Constricted Artery

Hamilton, R. W., Holling, H.E., and Roberts, B.: Relation of Pressure flow, and lumen during local arterial constriction. Surg. Forum., *14*:418, 1963.

Mann, F.C., Herrick, J.F., Essex, H.E., and Baldes E.J.: Effect on blood flow of decreasing the lumen of the blood vessel. Surgery, *4*:249, 1938.

Schultz, R.D., Hokanson, D.E. and Strandness, D.E., Jr.: Pressure flow relations and stress—strain measurements of normal and diseased aorto-iliac segments. Surg., Gyn., Obstet., *124*:1267, 1966.

Collateral Flow

John, H.T. and Warren, R.: The stimulus to collateral circulation. Surgery, *49*:14, 1961.

Ludbrook, J.: Collateral artery resistance in the human lower limb. J. Surg. Res., *6*:423, 1966.

Cranley, J.J., Hermann, L.G. and Preuninger, R.M.: Evaluation of factors which influence the circulation of extremities with obliterative vascular disease. Surgery, *34*:1076, 1953.

Reivich, M., Holling, H.E., Roberts, B., and Toole, J.F.: Reversal of blood flow through the vertebral artery and its effect on the cerebral circulation. New Eng. J. Med., *265*:878, 1961.

Roberts, B., Hardesty, W., Holling, H. E., Reivich, M., and Toole, J.: Studies on extracranial cerebral blood flow. Surgery, *56*:826, 1964.

Effect of Body Heating on Blood Flow to Digits

Gibbon, J.M., Jr. and Landis, E.M.: Vasodilatation in the lower extremities in response to immersing the forearms in warm water. J. Clin. Invest., *11*:1019, 1932.

Lewis, T. and Pickering, G.W.: Vasodilation in the limbs in response to warming the body: with evidence for sympathetic vasodilator nerves in man. Heart, *16*:33, 1931.

Effect of Body Heating on Blood Flow to Skin of more Proximal Portions of Limbs

Fox, R.H. and Hilton, S.M.: Bradykinin formation in human skin as a factor in heat vasodilatation. J. Physiol., *142*:219, 1958.

Grant, R.T. and Holling, H.E.: Further observations on the vascular responses of the human limb to body warming: evidence for sympathetic vasodilator nerves in the nomal subject. Clin. Sci., *3*:273, 1938.

Roddie, I.C., Shepherd, J.T. and Whelan, R.F.: The contribution of constrictor and dilator nerves to the skin vasodilatation during body heating. J. Physiol., *136*:489, 1957.

Effect of Temperature on Blood Flow Through Muscle

Barcroft, H. and Edholm, O.G.: Temperature and blood flow in the human forearm. J. Physiol., *104*:366, 1946.

Effect of Lowered Perfusion Pressure on Blood Through Muscle

Burton, A.C. and Yamada, S.: Relation between blood pressure and flow in the human forearm. J. Appl. Physiol., *4*:329, 1951.

Holling, H.E. and Verel, D.: Circulation in the elevated forearm. Clin. Sci., *16*:197, 1957.

Holling, H.E., Boland, H.C., and Russ, E.: Investigation of arterial obstruction using a mercury in rubber strain gauge. Amer. Heart Journ., *62*:194, 1961.

Sympathetic Innervation of Vessels Supplying Voluntary Muscle

Barcroft, H., Bonnar, W. Mck., Edholm, O..G. and Effron, A.S.: On sympathetic vasoconstrictor time in human skeletal muscle. J. Physiol., *102*:21, 1943.

Barcroft, H., Brod, J., Hejl, Z., Hirsjarvi, E.A. and Kitchin, A.H.: The mechanism of the vasodilatation in the forearm muscle during stress (Mental Arithmetic). Clin. Sci., *19*:577, 1960.

Blair, D.A., Glover, W.E., Greenfield, A.D.M. and Roddie, I.C.: Excitation of cholinergic vasodilator nerves to human skeletal muscles during emotional stress. J. Physiol., *148*:633, 1959.

Brigden, W., Howarth, S., Scharpey-Schafer, E.P.: Postural changes in peripheral blood flow of normal subjects with observations on vasovagal fainting reactions as a result of tilting, the lordotic posture, pregnancy and spinal anesthesia. Clin. Sci., *9*:79, 1950.

Holling, H.E.: Effect of embarrassment on blood flow to skeletal muscle. Trans. of Amer. Clin. and Climat. Asso., *76*:49, 1965.

The Action of Humoral Agents on Blood Flow to Muscle

Holling, H.E.: Observations on the oxygen content of venous blood from the arm vein and on the oxygen consumption of resting human muscle. Clin. Sci., *4*:103, 1939.

Patterson, G.C. and Shepherd, J.T.: The effects of continuous infusions into the brachial artery of adenosin triphosphate, histamine and acetyl choline on the amount and rate of blood flow-debt repayment following rhythmic exercise of the forearm muscles. Clin. Sci., *13*:85, 1954.

Release of Tone in Resistance Vessels by Sympathectomy

Barcroft, H. and Walker, A.J.: Return on tone in blood vessels of the upper limb after sympathectomy. Lancet, *1*:1035, 1949.

Dornhorst, A.C., and Sharpey-Schafer, E.P.: Collateral resistance in limbs with arterial obstruction: spontaneous changes and effects of sympathectomy. Clin Sci., *10*:371, 1951.

Grant, R.T. and Holling, H.E.: Further observations on the vascular responses of the human limb to body warming; evidence for sympathetic vasodilator nerves in the normal subject. Clin. Sci., *3*:273, 1958.

Lynn, II.B. and Barcroft, H.: Circulatory changes in the foot after lumbar sympathectomy. Lancet, *1*:1105, 1950.

Trotter, W. and Davies, H.M.: Experimental studies in the innervation of the skin. J. Physiol., *38*:134, 1908-9.

Microcirculation

Ditzel, J.: Morphologic and Hemodynamic changes in the smaller blood vessels in diabetes mellitus. New Eng. J. Med., *250*:541, 1954.

Kuo, P.T., Feng, L.Y. and Pamintuan, J.: Studies of nailfold capillaries in hypertriglyceridemia. (Types III and IV hyperlipoproteinemia). Circ., *41*:309, 1970.

Weideman, M.P.: Dimensions of blood vessels from distributing artery to collecting vein. Circ. Res., *12*:375, 1963.

Wells, R.E.: Rheology of blood in the microvasculature. New Eng. J. Med., *270*:832, 1964.

Wells, R.E., Herman, M., and Gorlin, R.: Microvascular changes in coronary disease. Cir., *34*:237, 1967.

General Properties of Veins

Wood, J. Edwin: The Veins p. 224. Boston, Little Brown and Co., 1965.

————: Physiology of the Veins *in* Conn, H.L. and Horwitz, O. (eds.); Cardiac and Vascular Diseases. Philadelphia, Lea and Febiger, 1971.

Venous Valves

Beecher, H.K., Field, M.E. and Krogh, A.: The effect of walking on the venous pressure at the ankle. Skand Archiv J. Physiol., *73:* 133, 1936.

Holling, II.E., Beecher, H.K. and Linton, R.R.: Study of the tendency to edema formation associated with incompetence of the valves of the communicating veins of the legs. Oxygen tension of blood contained in varicose veins. J.C.I., *17*:555, 1938.

Effect of External Pressure on Venous Volume in a Limb

Wilkins, R.W., Mixler, G., Stanton, J.R. and Litter, J.: Elastic stockings in the prevention of pulmonary embolism. A preliminary report. New Eng. J. Med., *246*:360, 1952.

Lymphatic System

Borodin, Y.I. and Tomchik, G.V.: Functional relationships between the blood vessels and lymphatic sinuses under normal conditions and during experimental disturbances of blood and lymph circulation. Byull. Eksp. Biol. Med., *60*:50, 1965.

Threefoot, S.A., et al.: Factors stimulating function of lymphaticovenous communications. Angiology, *18*:682, 1967.

Yoffey, J.M. and Courtice, F.C.: Lymphatics lymph and lymphmyeloid complex. New York, Academic Press, 1970.

2

Interview and Examination of a Patient with Arterial Disease

In this chapter an account is given of symptoms which may lead the physician to consider that his patient is suffering from arterial disease and the examinations which may be carried out to make a diagnosis. Guide lines for the questioning and examination of such a patient are listed below, and the outline is filled in in the following paragraphs.

EXAMINATION OF PATIENT WITH VASCULAR DISEASE

INTERVIEW	
General information:	Name, age and sex.
	Eating, smoking and drinking habits.
Complaint:	Character and localization. Intermittent or constant.
	What relieves and what provokes?
	If associated with walking, what distance, and how quickly does relief come with rest?
	Effect of dependency, temperature or medication. Is the skin more or less sensitive than normal?
Associated conditions:	Diabetes mellitus, heart disease; anemia or polycythemia; other systemic disorder; mechanical or thermal injury.

EXAMINATION	
Appearance:	Color, swollen or atrophied. Condition of nails. Ulceration. Thrombosis or dilatation of superficial veins.
Feel:	Temperature and tightness of skin. Sweating.

	Arterial pulses. Upper limb: carotid, subclavian, brachial, radial, ulnar, digital. Lower limb: aorta, femoral, popliteal, posterior tibial, dorsalis pedis.
Office tests:	Oscillometer, arterial pressure in limbs (use wide cuff for thighs). Reactive hyperemia. Tourniquet tests for venous incompetence.
Laboratory tests:	Skin temperature under controlled conditions. Blood flow measurements by plethysmograph, or uptake of tagged material from tissues. Volume pulse in limbs and arterial pressure gradient. Arteriography or venography.

INTERVIEW

Coldness of the Extremities

Many patients complain of coldness of their hands or feet, but few have organic arterial disease. An immobile limb is cold because it lacks the exothermic reaction of muscular activity which normally contributes to the heat of a limb; also, in the absence of activity the blood flow to the limb diminishes. Thus patients with organic paralysis (poliomyelitis) or functional paralysis (shoulder-hand syndrome) will complain of coldness, but their limbs become warm when they are in a warm environment. It is only when coldness of a limb persists in a warm environment that organic arterial obstruction should be suspected.

Numbness and Tingling

When numbness and tingling are the result of ischemia the degree of ischemia is severe and obvious and the symptom persistent. Patients with minor degrees of ischemia also may complain of numbness and tingling, but it is doubtful whether this symptom is caused by their disease. In diabetics, the symptom may be the result of neuritis, in others it may arise from lumbosacral disease. In the upper limb particularly, is the numbness and tingling associated with pressure on the nerves at the thoracic outlet misinterpreted as due to vascular insufficiency (See Chap. 8).

Intermittent Claudication

Pain in the muscles brought on by exercise and relieved by rest is the most frequent presenting sign of obstruction of the main arteries of the limbs, so that a physician begins to suspect that condition as soon as he is told of pain in the legs associated with exercise. The symptom is easy to produce in oneself, and every young physician should do so to fix its characteristics in his mind. It is possible to produce the symptom in the leg, but it is more convenient to do so in the arm. A cuff on the arm is rapidly inflated to a pressure well above systolic and then an object is strongly grasped at the rate of about one per second. After about 30 grasps a diffuse aching pain will be felt in the flexor muscles of the forearm and hand, and after another 30 grasps or so the pain will become intolerable. The pain continues even though the exercise is stopped until the circulation is restored, when it disappears promptly. Such a test demonstrates the following features of intermittent claudication:

1. No pain when the muscles are at rest.
2. Gradual onset of pain which becomes intolerable after a definite amount of exercise.
3. The pain is confined to ischemic muscles.
4. The pain disappears promptly when the blood flow is restored.
5. A reflex rise of pulse rate and blood pressure occurs with the pain of intermittent claudication, though this does not appear to have any recognized clinical significance.

Sometimes the pain is described as a cramp, but tonic muscular spasm (Charley horse) is seldom a feature of chronic arterial insufficiency.

An exact history of intermittent claudication in the diagnosis of arterial disease is of prime importance, whether for a positive or a negative diagnosis. If the patient is a poor historian, or the site or time of onset of the pain is unusual, it is helpful to walk with him as he provokes a bout of pain to observe the time of its onset, its location and the promptness of its relief on resting.

Intermittent claudication is usually classed as "1 block, 2 blocks, etc.," and this is a useful but very rough measure of its severity. It is true that the pain usually comes on after having walked a specific distance at a certain speed, but the pain may be brought on sooner if the pace is quickened, and if the pace is desultory with frequent rests no pain may arise. The following type of remark is typical of a patient with intermittent claudication: "I can walk around the plant all day without feeling it, but it always comes on when I walk from my office to the parking lot."

The location of the pain, and to some degree its character depend on the site of the arterial obstruction. The usual site of atheromatous block is in the superficial femoral artery, so the pain usually occurs in the calf muscles. When the arteries of the calves and feet are blocked, as in early thromboangiitis obliterans, intermittent claudication occurs in the intrinsic muscles of the feet; pain in the feet is usually considered to be due to an orthopedic problem, so the patient gets fitted with arch supports. When the terminal aorta and iliac arteries are obstructed (Leriche syndrome) intermittent claudication occurs in the muscles of the thighs and buttocks. Usually a pain comparable to that in the calves is complained of however, the discomfort may occur after an insignificant amount of exercise and though it is sufficient to stop the activity it is described as weakness or tiredness only. These patients are in danger of being misdiagnosed as having an orthopedic lesion of the lumbosacral region.

An unusual manifestation of intermittent claudication occurred in a patient with obstruction of the branches of the aortic arch (aortic arch syndrome or pulseless disease). She complained of tiredness of the temporal and masseter muscles on chewing her food. The symptom was relieved by an aortacarotid graft. Claudication in the masseters and temporal muscles has also been described in temporal arteritis.

A pedant would say that intermittent claudication (intermittent limping) should not be used to describe the symptoms in the arms, but usage permits this misnomer. For a number of reasons intermittent claudication seldom occurs in the upper extremities: These are:

1. Obliterative disease is less common in the arteries of the upper limbs.
2. The arms are seldom used for repetitive persistent movements.
3. On few occasions is there the need to persist in activity of the upper limbs as there is in walking.
4. Intermittent claudication in the arms may present as tiredness and is then not recognized as the pain of ischemia.

Rest Pain

With more severe ischemia the nutrition of the resting tissues is affected. The patient begins to suffer pain in his toes, or fingers, which prevents him sleeping. Sooner or later he learns that the pain in his toes is somewhat relieved by sitting with his legs dependent, so he spends his nights in a chair. The mechanism of this relief is that the arterial perfusion pressure in the feet when sitting is increased by the hydrostatic pressure of the difference in levels of his heart and his feet, but since the venous pressure is likewise increased, edema is likely to form.

Ulceration

Ulcerations on hands and feet caused by ischemia is intensely painful. If a patient's feet are ulcerated and he does not complain of pain, the most likely cause of his lesion is diabetic neuropathy.

Impotence

The symptom of sexual impotence in the male comes first to the mind of a medical student when asked of the features of aortoiliac obstruction (Leriche syndrome). It is true that this symptom is described in Leriche's description, but in this country and in Britain it does not appear to be the practice of physicians to inquire specifically into this symptom. There were a number of reasons for this omission: one was the reticence of an older generation to discuss sexual matters, another was that little is known and little has been written on the physical causes of failure to maintain an erection, but mostly the reticence sprang from the realization that the possibility of restoration of potency following arterial surgery was uncertain even if the arterial stenosis was corrected. The franker approach of the present generation to sexual matters provides sounder information and an improvement in treatment (See Chap. 4, pp. 84, 85).

EXAMINATION

Skin Temperature and Color

Examination of a patient for arterial disease should be done in warm and comfortable surroundings, for even a healthy person who is cold and apprehensive is likely to have peripheral vaso-constriction. In white races the color of the skin is chiefly derived from blood in the subcutaneous venous plexus, and reduction of blood flow through the skin results in pallor or cyanosis. Pallor occurs when the vessels of the microcirculation are constricted, and cyanosis occurs when the venules are dilated. To place much significance on minor degrees of pallor or cyanosis may be misleading because blood flow through the skin is greatly affected by environmental temperature. However, if the change is definite, particularly if it is localized to a digit, or a hand, or a foot so that comparison can be made with the normal skin color, the sign becomes one of great value. Elevation of the limb above heart level will intensify pallor in an ischemic limb, whereas the color of the limb with normal circulation will not be affected. Pallor of the feet may also be intensified after walking. In these circumstances the vasodilatation in the active muscles "steals" blood which would otherwise reach the skin of the feet (Fig. 2-1).

With severe ischemia the skin of the feet is often bright red (rubor) when the leg is dependent and pallid when it is elevated. According to Sir Thomas Lewis, the redness, indicating oxyhemo-globin in the corpuscles, persists because the tissues are so cold

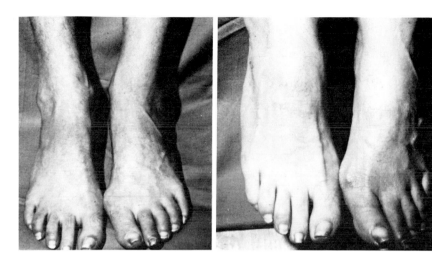

Fig. 2-1. Patient with more severe vascular disease in the right leg than in the left. Pallor developed in the right foot after the patient had walked up and down the hospital corridor.

that the skin cannot readily take up, nor the hemoglobin give up, its oxygen. These color changes are appreciated with greater difficulty in nonwhite patients, especially since I have observed a deepening of the melanotic pigmentation in the foot affected with unilateral vascular disease.

Chronic ischemia results in atrophic changes in the skin so that it appears shiny and tightly drawn over the underlying tissues. The pulp or pad of the terminal phalanx of the digits atrophies and the hardened skin over it can be dented in in the manner of a table tennis ball. The nails become thickened and hardened, epithelial debris accumulates under their edges and lesions around them fail to heal. As a result of these changes the cutaneous hair fails to grow, but the distribution of hair on the limbs varies so much from person to person that its presence or absence seems hardly worthy of notice.

Correct interpretation of small but significant differences in skin temperature as detected by hand requires more experience and skill than is generally realized. The limbs should have been exposed and at rest for at least 10 minutes and the skin temperatures of one limb should be checked and rechecked with those of the other at a similar location before any pronouncement is made. Under cool conditions the limbs are cooler than the trunk, the legs and feet cooler than the arms and hands, and the skin temperature decreases steadily to the fingers and toes. Thus the temperature of the digits provides a good indication of the state of the circulation to the whole limb. However, when the subject becomes warm the arteriolovenous anastomoses of his digits open up (See Chap. 8) and under these circumstances the temperature of his digits may be higher than that of the more proximal parts of his limbs. Knowing these facts, it will be appreciated that a more significant observation is when one limb or portion of one limb is found to have a temperature different from that of the comparable area on the opposite limb.

Localized Ischemia

Ischemia of an extremity is usually general, but the physician should be alert to recognize localized ischemia when it results from showers of small emboli. Figure 2-2 shows spotty patches of persistent cyanosis on one foot. In this case the condition followed immediately on arterial reconstruction and was presumed due to dislodgement of small plaques of atheroma at the site of the operation. A more usual cause for patchy ischemia in one foot, or leg is showers of emboli from a popliteal aneurysm. The same condition in the fingers is likely to be due to emboli from a subclavian aneurysm, or to digital artery thrombosis (See Chap. 8).

Peripheral Pulses

The quality of pulsation in the peripheral arteries provides the means of determining the location of arterial obstruction at the bedside. The value of combining auscultation of the major arteries with palpation of their pulsation has been recognized; still to be appreciated is the form of the pulse, for distal to a stenosis the pulse may be expected to be slow rising as well as being of low amplitude. Refinement of technique of bedside examination of

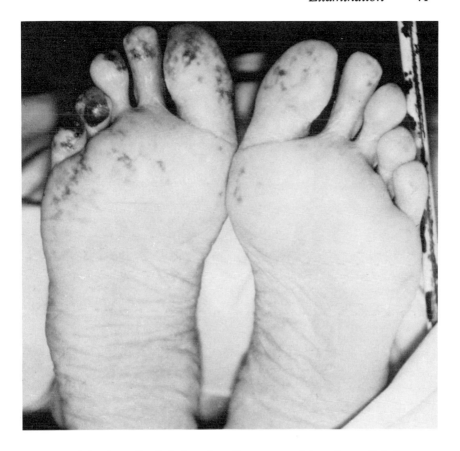

Fig. 2-2. Localized ischemia of toes resulting from "cholesterol" or "atheromatous" emboli dislodged during aortoiliac
reconstruction.

the arterial system is a worthwhile ambition, for precision in
localizing the site of arterial obstruction is the big first step in the
differential diagnosis of arterial disease. It is true that arteriography will localize the obstruction more precisely, but unless
the physician bases his directions for arteriography on a thorough
bedside examination he will occasionally be guilty of requesting
arteriography on the wrong area.

Peripheral pulsation is of less value as an indication of the adequacy of blood flow to the tissues; examples are: (1) the radial pulse in an elevated arm feels stronger, being more collapsing, but the blood flow to the hand is diminished; (2) in phlegmasia cerulea dolens the peripheral pulses are bounding, but the distal tissues are ischemic because the microcirculation is thrombosed; (3) there may be no femoral or popliteal pulse in cases of long-standing obstruction of iliac and femoral vessels, but a network of collateral vessels provides an adequate blood supply to the tissues.

The art of palpation of pulses is one to be learned at the bedside; the words of Paracelsus: "not even a dog killer can learn his trade from books, but only from experience, and how much more is this true of the physician." The following notes are offered to supplement bedside learning.

At times the physician has to question whether the pulse he is feeling is that of the patient or the pulsation in his own finger tips. The simplest means of distinguishing is to palpate about 1 cm. laterally with the same firmness; if the pulse felt was the patient's it will no longer be palpable, whereas it will still be appreciable if it was that of the observer.

Carotid Pulse. If the artery is tucked away behind the sternomastoid muscle, its pulsation may be felt only with deep probing. Make a habit of routinely palpating the superficial temporal artery, which requires only light palpation. Prominent carotid pulsation is more likely to be the result of tortuosity of the vessel than due to an aneurysm. Since the most frequent site for atherosclerotic stenosis is at the origin of the internal carotid which lies high in the neck, behind the angle of the jaw, it is here that the systolic bruit of stenosis of the internal carotid is to be sought. Systolic murmurs in the common carotid must be traced towards the heart in case they are the transmitted murmur of aortic stenosis. Palpation of the internal carotid pulse in the tonsillar fossa is an unrewarding procedure, and measurement of the retinal artery pressure is a better way of assessing the degree of obstruction of the internal carotid.

Subclavian Artery. This artery is usually down behind the clavicle, but with abnormalities of the thoracic outlet the vessel may be pushed up so that its pulsation is to be felt above the clavicle. In this case auscultation about the clavicle should be carried out as the arm is moved into different positions. Subclavian obstruction with a possible "subclavian steal" may be detected by the bruit at the base of the neck with a reduction of brachial pressure in the left arm and a reduction in amplitude of the radial pulse.

Axillary and Brachial Arteries. In cases of embolism the site of lodgement in these vessels may be felt.

Radial Artery. It takes less time to feel both radial arteries simultaneously, and this is likely to be more informative when there is a difference in arterial supply to the two arms.

Ulnar Artery. When this artery lies beneath the flexor carpi ulnaris tendon the wrist must be flexed and the tendon pushed medially before the arterial pulsation can be felt. Arteriography of the upper limb seems to show an undue number of cases in which the ulnar artery is lacking at the wrist. These findings and the use of the Allen test in assessing the contribution of the radial and ulnar arteries to the blood supply of the hand are discussed in Chapter 8.

Digital Pulses. Thorough examination of a patient with digital ischemia may require examination of the digital pulses. These are to be felt at the base of each side of the digit, preferably after the hand has been warmed by soaking in warm to hot water.

Femoral Pulse. A careful assessment of the quality of the femoral pulse is required to decide whether a patient is to have a simple femoral arteriogram or the more complicated procedure of an aortogram. The question to be asked is whether there is any indication of obstruction in the terminal aorta or iliac vessels. Indications of such obstruction are a difference in force of the two femoral vessels, a slow rising and low amplitude pulsation, and the presence of a systolic bruit over the vessel. Auscultation should be extended up into the abdomen and down along the line of the adductor canal. If obstruction is suspected very useful information is provided by measurement of the arterial pressure in the legs. In the older male patient the diameter of the artery should be noted as an indication of medial arteriosclerosis which is associated with widening of the arteries and aneurysmal formation. The thrombosed artery may be felt as a firm cord, again palpation down the adductor canal may reveal the length of the thrombosis.

Popliteal Artery. It is important to become competent in assessing the quality of the popliteal pulse. Distal ischemia associated with a palpable popliteal pulse implies that arterial surgery is unlikely to be feasible. Absence of the pulse implies superior femoral block, which can probably be relieved by surgery.

To feel the popliteal pulse well, have the patient lie prone with his knees flexed at a right angle and all his muscles relaxed. Using the finger tips of both hands and pressing firmly feel the midline of the popliteal fossa from top to bottom. If the pulsation can be felt with both hands when the hands are slightly separated the presence of a popliteal aneurysm must be suspected. When the lower part of the superficial femoral artery and the popliteal is blocked no popliteal pulsation can be felt, but light palpation at each side of the knee may give the observer the satisfaction of feeling the lateral and medial geniculate arterial pulsations, for these provide the collateral circulation.

Dorsalis Pedis and Posterior Tibial Pulses. The location of these pulses varies slightly from patient to patient, particularly the dorsalis pedis pulse. In a survey of 360 medical students Dr. Horwitz and I found the dorsalis pedis pulses to be absent in only one. The development of collateral circulation with a high (iliac) obstruction is often so good that the pulses of the feet are often palpable even though more proximal pulses are absent.

Arterial Pressures

Measurement of arterial pressure distal to an obstruction gives a very good estimation of the effect of the obstruction, for the pressure measured represents the balance of the effect of the stenosis in reducing distal pressure and of collateral circulation in maintaining it.

Retinal artery pressure, measured by ophthalmodynamometer, should be routine procedure in all patients suspects of carotid artery stenosis.

Brachial artery pressures should be measured in both arms in all routine physical examinations and *must* be compared when simultaneous palpation of the radial pulses suggests arterial obstruction in one arm. A difference of systolic pressure of more than 20 mm. Hg indicates significant stenosis; if the difference is less than this, it is advisable to enlist the aid of an associate so that the pressure in both arms can be measured simultaneously. This eliminates the possibility that differences found are the result of fluctuations in aortic pressure. Measurement of brachial artery pressure with the arm in different positions may be used to give a measure of the degree of arterial obstruction occurring in patients with thoracic outlet syndrome, not forgetting that allowance for hydrostatic pressure difference must be made when the arm is lifted above heart level.

Femoral artery pressure measurement requires the use of a thigh cuff of at least 17 cm. in width. A Velcro fastening is usually found to be unsatisfactory for this cuff, and the bandage provided instead should be of length sufficient that it remains in position when the cuff is inflated. In addition, some means of monitoring distal blood flow as the cuff is inflated and deflated is required. Korotkoff sounds in the popliteal space are the usual method, but this is seldom feasible when vascular disease exists. A proportion of patients with aortoiliac obstruction retain a dorsalis pedis pulse. When present, it can be used, for though only systolic pressure can be detected, this is enough to show the severity of the obstruction. In the absence of palpable distal arterial pulsation the pressure can still be measured, though the apparatus used is less frequently available. It has been said that the oscillometer can be used for this purpose, but I have not taken the opportunity to test this out. Both Strandness and I have used the mercury in rubber strain gauge to detect distal flow, but the apparatus required makes this a laboratory rather than a bedside procedure. It seems likely that the transcutaneous ultrasonic flow detector could be employed usefully for this purpose.

DIAGNOSTIC TESTS

Allen's Test

This test for the circulation of the hand is a useful one. The observer compresses both radial and ulnar arteries at the patient's wrist and asks him to raise his hand and open and close his fist a few times to drive blood out of the palmar skin. The hand is then lowered and one of the arteries released. Prompt flushing of the hand is an indication that the artery which has been released contributes normally to the circulation of the hand, faint flushing and delay of more than 5 seconds is an indication that the artery is obstructed, faint and delayed flushing to one or another digit indicates local arterial disease.

Adson's Maneuver

When Adson described this maneuver his intent was to describe a test which would indicate compression of the subclavian artery by the scalenus anticus muscle. Since that time compression of the artery by other structures at the thoracic outlet has been recognized, and I have extended the term Adson's maneuver to investigation of the effect on the radial pulse of different positions of the shoulder girdle relative to the rib cage.

Whilst feeling the radial pulse have the patient take a deep breath, brace his shoulders back, then turn his head first to one side and then to the other. The arm may then be abducted to the level of, and above, the shoulder (hyperabduction syndrome), then pulled downward at the elbow against the resistance of the patient. Note should be taken when the above positions result in obliteration of the pulse, and the maneuver should be repeated whilst listening for vascular bruits at the base of the neck. Disappearance of the pulse in one or other position is not necessarily abnormal, the findings should be weighed against the conditions under which the patient has symptoms. If the patient is to undergo arteriography the results of this test should be made known to the radiographer so that he may reproduce the position during arteriography.

Reactive Hyperemia

When blood flow is arrested metabolites accumulate in the tissues and result in relaxation of the tone of the small blood vessels. As circulation is restored the vasodilatation results in a greatly increased flow of blood. Observation of the degree and distribution of the hyperemia is used to indicate the extent of the arterial disease.

Allen's test, just described, is one form of reactive hyperemia test. In the classical test the limb should be kept warm, if necessary by immersion in water. It is then raised above heart level and may be massaged to drive blood out of the skin. The local circulation is then arrested by inflating a cuff on the limb to a pressure above systolic. The arrest is maintained for 5 to 10 minutes whilst the limb is kept comfortably warm. On release of the cuff the flush of reactive hypermia passes over the limb; with normal circulation the toes or fingers flush within less than 10 seconds, if there is organic arterial obstruction the flush is weakened and delayed. In this simple form the test has not come into wide use, one reason is that compression of the thigh by a pressure more than systolic is very uncomfortable. The test can be made quantitative and informative of the circulation to the deep tissues by using a plethysmograph to measure the reactive hyperemia.

INSTRUMENTAL DIAGNOSTIC TECHNIQUES

Oscillometry

The oscillometer provides an objective record of the arterial pulsation in a limb. When a pneumatic cuff is inflated on a limb to pressures between systolic and diastolic, the systolic thrust of blood flow under the cuff compresses the air in the cuff and the amplitude of compression can be recorded by suitable means. The effect of these systolic thrusts is seen in the small oscillations of the mercury column, or the deflections of the needle of an aneroid manometer when the blood pressure is measured. An oscillometer is in fact an aneroid manometer with a sensitive diaphragm which is attached to a blood pressure cuff. The cuff is inflated to a pressure well above systolic and reduced in steps of 10 mm. Hg at some point between systolic and diastolic pressure, a maximum excursion of the needle occurs and this is recorded. Different instruments differ in their sensitivity so that results obtained by different instruments can be compared only in a broad sense. This is shown by the wide range of oscillometer readings which are considered as normal:

	LOWER EXTREMITY		UPPER EXTREMITY
Thigh	8 to 15	Arm	5 to 12
Calf	4 to 10	Forearm	3 to 10
Ankle	1 to 5	Wrist	1 to 5

The oscillometer is useful to compare the pulsation in two limbs and produce an objective measurement. In cases of embolism the level on the limb at which pulsations abruptly stop may be determined.

Skin Temperature and the Vasodilation Test

In a steady state the surface temperature of the skin is somewhere between that of the superficial layer of the skin and the surrounding air. The temperature of the superficial layer is influenced by many factors. It depends on the rate of blood flow through the skin and the temperature of the arterial blood as it reaches the skin. It is affected by the evaporation of sensible and insensible perspiration and this in turn depends on the moistness of the skin and the dryness and rate of movement of the surrounding air. The skin is also warmed by blood flowing through underlying muscles and exothermic reactions taking place in them; in more proximal parts of the limb the skin may be warmed by warmer blood returning in the superficial veins.

Clearly skin temperature is not a reliable index of cutaneous blood flow, though it can be used as such under certain restricted conditions. The digits, being at the extremity of a limb, are not influenced by some of the factors which affect more proximal parts of the limb, moreover their circulation is specialized (see Chap. 8) to permit a wide range of blood flow so that their temperature can vary from that of room air to nearly that of the core of the body. Because of these facts the surface temperature of the fingers gives a better indication of blood flow through the skin than does the surface temperature of other parts of the body.

We have used thermocouples to measure the surface temperature of the digits in a room with controlled air temperature of 20 ±1°C. to standardize environmental conditions. To find the maximum blood flow which the circulation can supply to the digits, the vasoconstrictor effect of the sympathetic nervous system is removed by warming the patient strongly with heating pads, the feet or hands only being exposed to the cool air of the room. The skin temperature recorded under these conditions gives an indication of the severity of circulatory impairment, and whether there is adequate blood flow to the digits to supply their nutritional requirements. In practice the relationship which has been observed between the skin temperature of the digits at full dilatation and the adequacy of the circulation to them is given in Table 2-1.

TABLE 2-1. RELATION BETWEEN MAXIMUM SKIN TEMPERATURE
AND STATE OF CIRCULATION

State of Circulation	Temperature °C		
	Fingers		Toes
Normal	Above 32		Above 30
Reduced but adequate		Above 28	
Intermediate		25 to 28	
Very seriously reduced		Below 25	

This test was originally introduced as a means of foretelling the probable effect of sympathectomy. It is still used for that purpose, but its main use now is to give an objective measure of the circulation in order to indicate the urgency of arterial repair. The test may also be used to show absence of organic circulatory disease, as in a person with Raynaud's phenomenon, though at the higher rates of blood flow, that is between 40 and 100 ml./100 ml./min., the skin temperature is little affected by large increments in blood flow so that small degrees of impairment may be missed.

Another technique which has been used to record skin temperature is thermography. The heat radiated from the surface of the skin is picked up by an infrared thermistor which produces voltage differences proportional to surface temperature. The record is a photographic one which shows cooler areas in darker tones.

Plethysmography

Any instrument which is used to measure volume or change in volume is a plethysmograph and with intermittent venous occlusion can be used to measure blood flow in the limbs. Of the many types of plethysmograph I have used only the water-filled and the mercury in rubber (Whitney) strain gauge. The former is somewhat cumbersome for clinical use, the latter has the advantage of being easily applied and can be used at the bedside. Measurement of blood flow to a limb at rest does not, however, give a useful assessment of the circulation to a limb; for this purpose stress should be put on to the circulation either by exercising the muscles, or by observing the hyperemia which follows a period of vascular occlusion (reactive hyperemia). Neither test has come into general use. Both Strandness and I have found the strain gauge useful clinically in measurement of the arterial gradient in a limb to indicate the location and severity of an obstruction. The strain gauge might also be useful for measurement of the volume pulse for, particularly in the fingers, the amplitude of the volume pulse has been found to be proportional to the blood flow.

Transcutaneous Ultrasonic Doppler Flow Detectors

Flow velocity probes developed in recent years contain a sender and receiver of ultrasonic energy. Energy which is reflected back from moving surfaces is altered in frequency in proportion to the velocity of the moving surface (Doppler effect) so that the difference in frequency between the energy sent and the energy received is a measure of the velocity of the moving stream. The probe is placed on the skin over the blood vessel to be tested and as the energy impinges on the blood stream, some is reflected back into the probe. The frequency difference between emission and reception can be transmitted as sound within the audible range, or recorded by use of an analogue output that is proportional to the mean frequency of the audible signal.

It is difficult to calibrate this instrument exactly because some shift of frequency results from changes in the angle of incidence at which the energy strikes the blood stream. In spite of this limitation, the Doppler instrument appears to be useful for investigation of arterial obstruction and venous incompetence. It is particularly useful in that it can be taken to the bedside. Over the stenosis of an artery the flow detector shows a greater difference in frequency corresponding to the greater velocity of flow through the stenosis. No sound returns from an occluded artery. Over flowing venous blood a continuous sound signal is heard which can be augmented by distal compression of the limb squeezing more blood along the vein; also, the flow of the blood through an incompetent valve can be detected.

Impedance Plethysmography

Blood conducts electricity more easily than other tissues, so that impedance to the passage of an electric current through a portion of a limb varies with the proportion of blood in the tissue in circuit. Impedance of current is high in an ischemic limb and low in a plethoric limb. Sensitive and quickly responding apparatus has been developed which shows the changes in blood content of tissues through the pulse cycle. The source of the current is a battery, and an oscillator converts the direct current to a high frequency (30 to 50 kHz) current with a strength of less than 1 Ma. The frequency is too high to stimulate the heart, and the current strength is too low to be perceived by the patient. The current source is held constant and changes in voltage reflect changes in impedance, which in turn reflect changes in blood volume.

The apparatus is being used to measure pulsatile arterial flow. It has also been used to measure the changes in venous volume of the legs during deep inspiration and so indicate the presence or absence of deep vein thrombosis.

Radiologic Techniques

Straight radiography is particularly valuable in cases of aneurysm of the abdominal aorta in showing the calcification in the wall of the aneurysm. It is a noninvasive technique and in the lateral view is a valuable step in diagnosis of the condition, in observation of its progress, and in deciding whether surgical treatment is required. It is of less value in investigation of arterial disease of the limbs. Calcification of the vessels may be demonstrated, but this is seldom of diagnostic importance. In atherosclerosis, calcified plaques may be shown, but their discovery is seldom helpful, and the extensive calcification of medial calcification (Mönckeberg's sclerosis) does not result in arterial obstruction.

Arteriography is particularly useful. The examination of a patient should aim to define the location and extent of the arterial disease so that if arteriography is required the physician may best advise the radiologist which particular study is required. By demonstration of the location and extent of the disease, and whether the vessels are affected segmentally as in atheroma or embolic obstruction, or along their length as in thromboangiitis obliterans, the presence of small aneurysms as in polyarteritis nodosa arteriography is valuable in the diagnosis of arterial disease. More extensive use of arteriography in the study of vascular diseases of the limbs is desirable.

GUIDELINES IN THE DIFFERENTIAL DIAGNOSIS OF ARTERIAL DISEASE

The age and sex of a patient and the localization of his arterial disease are very informative in differential diagnosis (Table 2-2 and Fig. 2-3). In some instances age, sex and localization of an arterial disease seem so specific that they raise hopes that these findings could be informative in the question of causation of disease, but so far this hope has not been realized.

TABLE 2-2. AGE, SEX AND LOCATION OF LESIONS IN ARTERIAL DISEASE

DISEASE	THROMBOANGIITIS OBLITERANS	COLLAGEN DISEASES	ATHEROSCLEROSIS WITH DIABETES	ATHEROSCLEROSIS	MEDIAL ARTERIOSCLEROSIS
AGE OF ONSET	20 TO 35	20 TO 50	40 TO 60	50 TO 60	OVER 60 YEARS
SEX	MALE	(SEE TEXT)	FEMALE > MALE	MALE:FEMALE = 6:1	MALE:FEMALE = 8:1
UPPER LIMB					
Subclavian artery	0	0	0	+	0
Radial and ulnar	++	+	0	0	0
Digital	+++	+++	0	0	0
ABDOMINAL AORTA					
AORTA ILIAC	0	0	0	+	+++
	0	0	+	++	+++
LOWER LIMB					
Femoral popliteal	0	0	+++	+++	++
Tibioperoneal	+++	0	+++	+	0
Digital	+++	+++	0	0	0

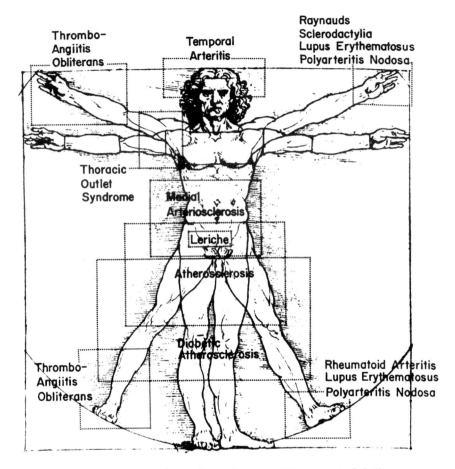

Fig. 2-3. Location of arterial lesions in different arterial diseases.

Age

Raynaud's phenomenon and lymphedema both characteristically appear with puberty. Thromboangiitis has its major effect in the prime of life, that is, in the fourth decade, but with earlier appearance in the twenties and lingering effects in the forties. It is unusual for the most prevalent arterial disease—atherosclerosis obliterans—to give rise to symptoms before the patient is 40 years old, even if the patient is diabetic. It is unusual for medial arteriosclerosis to result in an aneurysm of the aorta before the age of 60. The collagen diseases appear at any time over the wide span of a lifetime.

Sex

If you diagnose thromboangiitis in a female you are almost certain to be in error. Females in the childbearing period very seldom suffer from the effects of atherosclerosis obliterans, even if they are diabetic. Abdominal aneurysm due to medial atherosclerosis is ten times more common in old men than in old women. Polyarteritis nodosa is three times more common in males than in females, systemic lupus erythematosus is four times more common in females than in males, and scleroderma affects the sexes equally. Some textbooks state that Raynaud's phenomenon is five times more common in females than in males but give no basis for this statement. In practice more males than females are referred to consultants in vascular diseases, because the primary physician has been taught that Raynaud's phenomenon in a male may be of sinister import. In my experience Raynaud's phenomenon, that is, transient attacks of pallor and coldness of the fingers, occurs as frequently in men as in women. But Raynaud's disease, that is, more persistent coldness of the fingers leading to nutritional changes in them, is much more common in women. When persistent digital ischemia does occur in a man it is usually severe leading to necrosis of the fingers and due to organic arterial obstruction.

Localization

Two arterial diseases are remarkable in that they occur predominantly in specific arteries: temporal arteritis in the temporal arteries, and fibromuscular dysplasia in the renal arteries. These disorders are not confined to these arteries, but their main incidence is remarkably localized. Other arterial diseases tend to occur in particular locations but, as might be expected, they overspread fixed boundaries.

The occurrence of Raynaud's phenomenon in the digital arteries is not surprising in view of the extreme reactivity of those arteries; perhaps this explains too why, of peripheral arteries, the collagen diseases mainly attack these reactive vessels. Thromboangiitis obliterans affects medium sized and small arteries of the limbs, i.e., those distal to the elbow and knee, it does not affect visceral arteries including coronary and cerebral. Atherosclerosis has its major effect in the iliacfemoral arteries, it occurs seldom in the upper limb and not often below the popliteal unless the patient is diabetic. Medial arteriosclerosis is primarily a disease of the abdominal aorta below the renal arteries and extending into the iliac arteries.

REFERENCES

Holling, H.E., Boland, H.C., and Russ, E.: Investigation of arterial obstruction using a mercury in rubber strain gauge. Amer. Heart J., *62*:184, 1961.

Horwitz, O., and Abramson, D.G.: A modification of the vasodilatation test. Amer. J. Cardiol., *6*:663, 1960.

Strandness, D.E., Jr., and Bell, J.W.: Peripheral vascular disease: diagnosis and objective evaluation using a mercury strain gauge. Ann. Surg., [Suppl.] *161*:35, 1965.

Strandness, D.E., Jr., McCutcheon, E.P., and Rushmer, R.F.: Application of a trancutaneous Doppler flowmeter in evaluation of occlusive arterial disease. Surg. Gynec. Obstet., *122*:1039, 1966.

Wheeler, H.B., Mullick, S.C., Anderson, J.N., and Pearson, D.: Diagnosis of occult deep vein thrombosis by a non-invasive bedside technique. Surgery, *70*:20, 1971.

Part II

DISORDERS OF
LARGE ARTERIES

3

Acute Arterial Obstruction

ARTERIAL EMBOLUS

Major

A major embolus is one which lodges in the main artery to a limb: brachial, femoral, or in an artery proximal to that, including the bifurcation of the aorta.

The typical history is of an abrupt onset of pain and coldness in a limb. Venous thrombosis might also have an abrupt onset, but one is seldom confused with the other: distinguishing features are given in Table 3-1.

TABLE 3-1. COMPARISON OF ARTERIAL EMBOLISM
AND VENOUS THROMBOSIS

	EMBOLISM	THROMBOSIS
Pain	Severe and steady	Steady
Appearance of limb	Cold and pallid not swollen	Warm, cyanosed and swollen
Veins	Collapsed	Full
Pulsation	Absent	Present
Sensory and motor function	Diminished	No change

By careful palpation it is usually possible to determine the exact site of lodgement of the embolus, recognizing that it will lodge at the bifurcation of an artery. An important decision, and one that must be made early, is whether it is desirable to have the embolus removed by surgery. Within the past decade progress in vascular surgery has made embolectomy a safe and effective operation, and though prompt removal of the embolus is still desirable, progress in surgery has resulted in later removal being feasible. Even if a limb might survive the embolus, it is better that the limb should survive in a healthy state after removal of the embolus rather than that it should hang on in a state of chronic ischemia with its main artery of supply blocked. Routine pathological and bacteriological examination of the removed embolus may give the additional advantage of the diagnosis of an embolizing tumor, or an infected thrombus. However, the general state of the patient may defer an operative procedure, or the effectiveness of the collateral circulation may make embolectomy seem unnecessary.

Heparin therapy should be started as soon as possible to prevent propagation of the thrombus. Attendants should be warned against any attempt to warm up the limb by the application of direct heat because of the danger of burning the ischemic skin. If surgery is decided on, the patient should be removed to the place where this is carried out as soon as possible.

Minor

Minor emboli may be classed as those which lodge in the branches of the named arteries. These smaller emboli may originate in the heart, but often arise from the aorta and its branches.

Small areas of skin in the toes and sometimes the fingers are affected with the sudden onset of pallor or cyanosis, the lesions are usually tender and may be painful (Fig. 2-2). The tendency is for them to regress spontaneously, but they may coalesce and loss of tissues ensues or, as in cervical rib, repeated emboli may give rise to digital ischemia. Some ulcers of the shin, which are difficult to explain on arterial or venous etiologies may prove to be due to emboli from the aorta or iliac artery lodging in an end artery of the skin. The importance of minor emboli is that they should be recognized as such and their site of origin determined. The following possibilities must be considered:

Cardiac: bacterial endocarditis, mural thrombus from an infarct, atrial fibrillation, mitral stenosis, atrial myxoma, calcified aortic valve, artificial heart valve.

Aortic: atheroma, aneurysm.

Arterial: atheroma, trauma, arteriosclerotic or mycotic aneurysm, cervical rib or other thoracic outlet pressure.

Paradoxical Embolus

There is a cause of embolism which is more frequently spoken of than seen; this is the passage of an embolus from veins to artery through a patent foramen ovale. Because the usual direction of flow through a patent foramen ovale is from left to right atrium the so-called paradoxical embolus is a very rare occurrence and well named.

ARTERIAL THROMBOSIS

The local symptoms and signs in arterial thrombosis do not differ from those of embolus, but the general condition of most patients with thrombosis is likely to be poorer. This is one reason why surgical removal of the arterial obstruction is less often successful in thrombosis than in embolus; the other is that the condition underlying arterial thrombosis is likely to be irreversible. The predisposing conditions are listed below. When considering the prognosis of acute ischemia for life and limb the following factors are unfavorable: General: repeated emboli or thrombosis; heart failure; surgical or infective shock; cachexia; dehydration. Local: arteriosclerosis obliterans; aneurysm; increased metabolic demands of tissue by trauma or infection.

CONDITIONS PREDISPOSING TO ARTERIAL THROMBOSIS

STASIS
  Terminal cardiac failure and malignancy
  Gram negative bacteremia

HYPERCOAGULABILITY
  Polycythemia: rubra vera, secondary, and stress
  Thrombocytosis.
  Macroglobulinemia.
  Snake bite (Russell's viper and American copperhead)

LOCAL CONDITION
>   *Injury*
>   Iatrogenic: arterial puncture and catheterization, injection of irritant drugs
>   >   Trauma: Bruising, repeated compression by bone, muscle, or tendon
>   *Disease*
>   >   Atheroma, aneurysm, diseased arterial wall as in thromboangiitis obliterans and polyarteritis nodosa.

UNCERTAIN
>   Postpartum and postoperative states
>   Oral contraceptives
>   Homocystinuria

One cause of arterial thrombosis requires special mention because the need for prompt remedial action is imperative. This is the thrombosis which follows local arterial trauma—injury, arterial puncture and catheterization, or, even more serious, when an irritant substance (bromsulfalein, thiopentone) is injected into the brachial artery in error for the antecubital vein. The condition is serious because spasm of the artery intensifies the obstruction and affects the collateral circulation. Mild degrees of this mishap may pass off spontaneously, but very definite signs of improvement must be present before efforts to assist reestablishment of arterial flow are relaxed.

A heating pad or hotwater bottle may be placed over the antecubital fossa until surgical exposure can be done. The full length of the affected artery should be exposed and 2.5 per cent papaverine injected into and around the artery. Preparation for Mustard's maneuver should meantime be taking place. In this procedure the contracted artery is distended by forcible injection of warm saline into it through a fine needle. The maneuver is more likely to be successful if the proximal end of the contraction is first isolated between light bulldog clamps and dilatation effected in successive isolated section down the artery, allowing the arterial pulsation into each portion of the artery as it is opened up.

REFERENCES

Eastcott, H.H.G.: Arterial Surgery. pp. 235-255. Philadelphia, J.B. Lippincott, 1969.

Kinmonth, J.B., Hadfield, G.J. Connolly, J.E., Lee, R.H. and Amoroso, E.C.: Traumatic arterial spasm. Its relief in man and in monkeys. Brit. J. Surg., *44*:164, 1956.

Mustard, W.T. and Bull, C.: A reliable method for relief of traumatic vascular spasm. Ann. Surg., *155*:339, 1962.

4

Atherosclerosis Obliterans

Atherosclerosis obliterans is a disease of the arteries which affects middle-aged males and postmenopausal females predominantly. It results in an accumulation of lipoid material in the arterial lumen causing obstruction of the vessel directly, and sometimes thrombosis occurs secondarily on the roughened intima.

In the past atherosclerosis obliterans has been confused with thromboangiitis obliterans, but the clinical distinction between the two diseases is clear (See Table 9-1). Another arterial disease which many still do not distinguish from atherosclerosis obliterans is medial arteriosclerosis, the distinction between the two diseases is set out in Table 5-1.

ETIOLOGY

The etiology of atherosclerosis obliterans can conveniently be considered under three headings: abnormalities of the blood; changes in metabolism and structure of the arterial wall; and stress of hemodynamic forces on the arterial wall.

Abnormalities of the Blood

A century ago cholesterol was found to be a major constituent of the atherosclerotic plaque, and many studies subsequently have shown a clear relationship between hyperlipidemia and an increased incidence of atherosclerosis. It is this association which at the present time gives the greatest hope for gaining control of atherosclerosis, and which is considered in greater detail later in this chapter.

The mechanism by which increased lipoproteins in the blood give rise to deposition of atheromatous plaques is not clear. One

65

hypothesis suggests that constituents of the plasma filter through the arterial wall from the lumen to the adventitial lymphatics, and during this process low density lipoproteins are deposited in the intima and myo-intimal layers of the arterial wall, as a precipitate might collect in the interstices of a filter paper.

Another hypothesis assigns an important role to aggregation of blood platelets on a damaged and roughened intima, followed by lipomatous changes as the platelets undergo degeneration; subsequently thrombi are likely to form on the degenerated platelets. This theory originated with Rokitansky and was restated by Duguid. Apart from the well known association of polycythemia vera, and particularly thrombocytosis, with manifestations of atherosclerosis, this theory has little support in clinical observations. The role of platelets may indeed be secondary if they aggregate on preformed atheromatous plaques and if thrombosis occurs subsequently on them. This sequence could equally well account for the increased manifestations of atheroma in polycythemia vera and thrombocytosis.

Changes in Metabolism and Structure of the Arterial Wall

Opinions are shifting from the theory that atheroma is deposited on the arterial wall by a passive infiltration. The suggestion has been made that patients with the metabolic disorder which gives rise to hyperlipidemia may have also a similar disorder of the cells of the arterial wall giving rise to a local accumulation of lipids. Whereat (1970) makes an impassioned plea for the recognition of the arterial wall "as an organ with multiple biochemical duties and capacities which it unfailingly carries out." He goes on to suggest that if a mitrochondrial enzyme of the intimal layers, reduced nicotinamide-adenine dinucleotide (N.A.D.H.), is less oxidized than usual, the rate of fatty acid synthesis is accelerated and its oxidation inhibited. Winegrad (1970) studied the changes which take place in the metabolism of the arterial wall when it is immersed in high concentration of glucose. He finds this change facilitates the activity of the enzyme aldose reductase and results in an increased concentration of sorbital, a polyol derivative of aldose sugars. For the present the role of such changes in metabolism of the arterial wall itself in the mechanism of atheromatous formation is not clear, but they open up an important new field for investigation.

Stress on the Arterial Wall

The arterial system may be thought of as a high pressure system in pliable tubes in an active body. Such a system is one which would be liable to local mechanical factors causing wear and tear because of which atheroma might develop. Thus atheroma is more developed in the larger vessels where stretch and tension within the arterial wall is greatest, or where repeated bending of a vessel occurs, as when flexion of the knee bends the popliteal artery. An explanation of why atheroma affects the lower rather than the upper extremity by this theory would be that in the upright position the arterial pressure in the legs is higher than that in the arms. This explanation fails to account for the experience that, in the absence of diabetes, atheroma is more developed in the femoropopliteal artery than in the peroneal and anterior and posterior tibial arteries where the hydrostatic increase in arterial pressure is even greater. Nor does it explain why femoropopliteal atheroma is associated with a high incidence of atherosclerosis in the cerebral circulation where hydrostatic forces would tend to reduce local arterial pressure.

EXACERBATION OF ATHEROSCLEROSIS BY OTHER DISEASES

Though the cause of atherosclerosis is still to be defined, it is well recognized that its progress is accelerated by the presence of other diseases.

Hyperlipoproteinemia

Five patterns (phenotypes) of lipoprotein increase account for most primary lipidemias, and four are associated with an increased incidence of peripheral vascular disease. Secondary hyperlipidemia, such as that due to hypothyroidism or diabetes mellitus, may also be a factor in the development of peripheral vascular disease, and its proper treatment is clearly that of the primary disease.

The types of primary hyperlipidemia as classified by Fredrickson are given in Table 4-1. Type I, in which the lipid abnormality is of increased chylomicra absorbed from the gut, is the only one which is not associated with an increased incidence of atherosclerosis. All types except IV are fat sensitive, though the clinical studies of Kuo have shown that 90 per cent of patients with hyperlipidemia have an exaggerated endogenous lipogenesis on ingestion of carbohydrate.

Elaborate investigation of the lipoprotein fractions is not required for clinical work. Kuo has described how naked eye inspection of plasma obtained in the postprandial state can be very informative, and when more definite distinctions are required Fredrickson has found that 96 per cent of cases of hyperlipidemia are differentiated by knowledge of the levels of serum cholesterol and triglycerides.

Investigations of the relationship between lipoproteinemia and atherosclerosis of the lower extremities are few compared to those of the coronary arteries. A probable reason for this disparity is that coronary artery disease is feared as a killing disease, whereas peripheral arterial disease is considered to be a maiming disease. A comparison of the parallel investigations, however, shows features of considerable theoretical and probable practical importance. This interest lies in the finding that the type of lipoproteinemia associated with coronary atherosclerosis may differ in some respects from that associated with peripheral arterial disease. Some studies suggest that patients with hypercholesterolemia (due to elevated plasma-β-lipoprotein levels) are more liable to coronary atherosclerosis than patients with hypertriglyceridemia, who in turn are more liable to atherosclerotic disease of the lower extremities. Workers who have participated in these investigations would agree that future studies should take advantage of the precise quantitative methods for measurements of lipoproteins, but there may be less awareness that advantage should also be taken of greater precision in the diagnosis of peripheral arterial

TABLE 4-1. TYPES OF PRIMARY HYPERLIPIDEMIA

TYPE	APPEARANCE OF PLASMA	CHOLESTEROL	TRIGLYCERIDES NORMAL RANGE	PHOSPHOLIPIDS
		160-260	50-150	6.5-12.5 MG./100 ML.
Non-carbohydrate Sensitive				
I	Milky	Normal	Increased	Chylomicra +
II (familial hypercholesterolemia)	Clear	Increased	Normal	β-lipoprotein increased
Carbohydrate Sensitive				
III	Turbid	Increased	Increased	Abnormal β-lipoproteins present
IV	Turbid	May be slight increase	Increased	Pre-β-lipoprotein increased
V	Milky	Increased	Increased	Chylomicra and pre-β-lipoprotein increased

disease. Physicians who are not particularly interested in vascular disease find it convenient to lump together all arterial disease in the older patient as "arteriosclerosis," but for the purpose of investigation greater precision in definition of the arterial disease should be attempted. It is already clear that factors which result in widening of the lumen of the abdominal aorta and iliac arteries ("arteriosclerotic aneurysm of the abdominal aorta") are likely to differ from those which result in blockage of the femoral artery by atheroma. There have also been suggestions that patients with obstruction of the terminal aorta and iliac arteries differ from those with arterial blocks predominantly in the femoral and sural arteries in that disorders of carbohydrate metabolism predominate in the latter group. The existence of other patterns of disease is certainly possible in the continuum of "atherosclerosis".

The question of whether reduction of hyperlipoproteinemia can result in halting of the atherosclerotic process is deferred to the section on consideration of the results of treatment.

Hypertension

It is usually assumed that the incidence of atheroma is greater in patients with hypertension, but it may be that the increased blood pressure augments the effects of existing atherosclerosis, even if it does not initiate the disease. There is little evidence on this point apart from the study of Roberts and his colleagues in 1959. They examined the arterial systems of 153 males who had died of atherosclerotic catastrophes. There was a more marked degree of coronary and cerebral arterial disease in those who had had arterial hypertension, and more evidence of myocardial infarcts. Another item which has been put forward in the argument for the importance of hypertension in the etiology of atheroma is the adverse effect of hypertension in patients with "arteriosclerotic aneurysm." The irrelevance of this fact will be shown in a later chapter where the use of the term "arteriosclerotic aneurysm" is deplored because the aneurysm is not the result of atherosclerosis but of a different disease: medial arteriosclerosis.

The question of whether hypertension exacerbates atheroma or rather exaggerates its effects has not been answered. Whatever the answer the practical question is whether control of hypertension diminishes the effects or retards the progress of atheroma. It is generally held that moderation of high blood pressure diminshes the incidence of vascular disease, meaning that a patient with controlled blood pressure can expect less congestive heart failure, cerebral hemorrhage, dissecting aneurysm and renal disease. Beneficial as these effects are, they could be ascribed to diminishing the consequences of atheroma, rather than to retarding its progress. In fact, Freis' careful study on the effect of controlling hypertension found that the incidence of myocardial infarcts was not reduced, suggesting that treatment of hypertension had not affected the progress of atheromatous disease. But even if the hypothesis that reduction of high blood pressure retards the development of atherosclerosis remains unproven, there is no doubt that its control may be expected to diminish the effects of the vascular disease.

Hyperglycemia

It has been said that when diabetes mellitus has been present for 20 years 92 per cent of patients show evidence of vascular disease, presumably atheroma. This is an oversimplification. There are at least two types of "diabetes mellitus" to be recognized. One, the "juvenile type" is usually diagnosed before middle age, the patient shows a tendency to ketosis and his hyperglycemia does not respond to oral agents; the other, diabetes of adult onset, manifests itself in middle age, the patients are not subject to ketosis and the hyperglycemia usually responds to oral agents. Atherosclerosis is associated with the diabetes of adult onset.

Patients with diabetes of the juvenile type succumb to renal disease or infection rather than to vascular disease. The lesions on the feet associated with the diabetic neuropathy have a very good blood supply. The arteriogram in Figure 4-1 shows the blood supply to a penetrating ulcer of the foot in a 42-year-old diabetic patient. The blood supply is so good that the term blush has been used to describe it. These patients were formerly described as having small vessel disease, i.e., a thickening of the intima of the small arteries, but this has not been found to be so in the observations of Strandness and his colleagues.

Patients with diabetes of adult onset are subject to exaggerated progress of atheroma in the coronary, cerebral and arteries of the lower extremities. In the lower extremities diabetes accelerates the progress of atheroma below the knee rather than above the

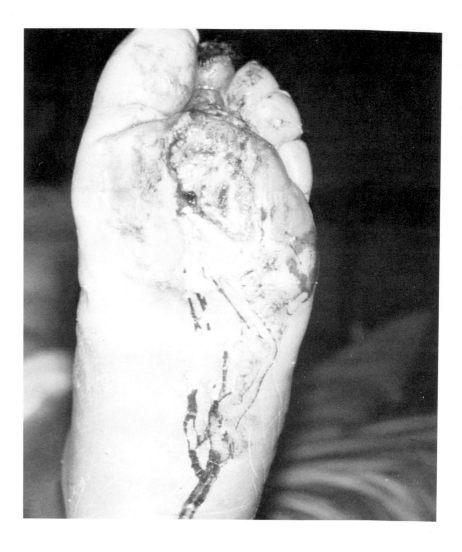

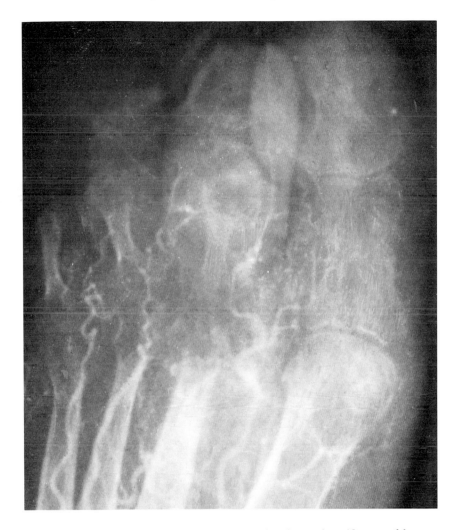

Fig. 4-1. (*Left*) Penetrating ulcer on the foot of a 42-year-old man with diabetic neuropathy. The good blood supply is shown by the exudate from the ulcer, by the bleeding which follows debridement, and by the arteriogram. The ulcer started when the man walked for some hours with a nail in his foot without feeling pain. (*Right*) X-ray of foot pictured above.

inguinal ligament. Thus we found no increased incidence of diabetes in a group of patients with aortoiliac obstruction (Leriche
syndrome), a greater than normal proportion of patients with
diabetes when the femoropopliteal artery was affected, and almost all patients were diabetic if tibial and peroneal arteries were
affected in addition to the femoral artery.

It has still not been decided if control of hyperglycemia in
patients with diabetes of adult onset, by diet, insulin, or by oral
agents, will retard the progress of atheroma. Of the many attempts to answer this question about half found that control of
hyperglycemia retards the progress of arterial disease; a third
find that control has no effect; others produce equivocal results.
One well publicized study suggested that control of hyperglycemia with an oral agent might increase the incidence of cardiovascular disease. Perhaps these divergent results could have been
forecast from the clinical observation that the severity of atherosclerosis in diabetes of adult onset is not related to the level of
the hyperglycemia, indicating that factors other than the level of
blood sugar are concerned in the development of atheroma.

Until this question is answered the best advice to offer seems
to be that the practitioner should hold to his belief that control
of hyperglycemia by one means or another must be to the advantage of his patient. The investigator might consider which
criterion should be used to monitor "control" of the diabetes;
perhaps control of the triglyceride level of the blood might be a
more effective means of retarding development of atherosclerosis.

Obesity

Obesity is associated with an increased incidence of both diabetes
and hypertension and it is consequently associated with an increased incidence of atheroma and its effects. However, the
Framingham Study found that obese subjects who were neither
diabetic nor hypertensive did not have an increased tendency to
atheroma as judged by the incidence of coronary, cerebral, or
peripheral vascular disease. Albrink may have an explanation of
this difference in her distinction of two types of fat men *: the

* Personal communication.

fat *thin* man and the fat *fat* man, the difference being whether obesity developed after the age of 25 or was present from boyhood. In the first group there is likely to be hyperglyceridemia and presumably an increase in atheroma.

The main point remains that obesity is ugly and a threat to well being, so that determined efforts should be made to treat it.

Sedentary Life

Kannel's observations on the risk of coronary heart disease in persons taking regular physical exercise indicate that the more sedentary a person is, the greater is the likelihood that he will die of a myocardial infarct. Comparable studies have not been made on the effects of exercise in atheroma of the lower extremities. Autopsy and epidemiological observations strongly suggest that physical activity protects, not so much against having coronary attacks, but rather against an attack being fatal. A likely explanation of these findings is that regular exercise promotes an effective collateral circulation, and there is good reason to believe that this should occur in the limb muscles as well as in the myocardium.

PREVENTION OF ATHEROSCLEROSIS

Not many years ago atherosclerosis was considered as a degenerative disease and there was a pessimistic attitude to the possibility of preventing or reversing its effects; it is now reasonable to take a more optimistic, and aggressive, attitude.

Possible Measures

Though we still lack proof of the effectiveness of measures taken to prevent atheroma, it is of interest to consider what steps might be advised to this end, and with what chance of success. A campaign to alter the American way of life sounds utopian, but schools, colleges and other educational institutions could encourage regular physical exercise and discourage overeating. The school bus and the candy store would be recognized as early induction into a life of sloth and gluttony. For adults voluntary restriction of the use of automobile and elevator would be encouraged, and a change in diet which would prefer seafood to steak, starches to sugars, and a limited intake of fat. Cigarette smoking and drinking alcohol would be discouraged. The chance of success of such a program in urban U.S.A. is very small indeed because it presents a series of restrictions. It might have some chance of being acted on if it could be presented in a more positive manner comparable to the schooling which led this group to add vitamins and food supplements to an already excessive diet.

The question becomes more realistic when a routine physical examination indicates that a person has become particularly prone to develop atherosclerosis. The following findings would suggest this: an increase in weight in adult life, a family history of cardiovascular disease, impaired glucose tolerance, or hyperlipidemia. In such circumstances advice can be given with more hope that it will be followed. The most important dietary advice is a restriction of caloric intake until an ideal body weight is attained. It is helpful to discuss the patient's eating habits with him and attempt to modify these rather than to impose an alien regimen on him. Recent publicity concerning the effects of exercise have prompted sedentary, overweight men to take up some form of physical exertion. Spasmodic jogging, and periodic visits to a health spa may be beneficial, but the effects of introducing more exercise into everyday life, such as walking to the store or railroad station, and never taking an elevator for less than three floors are likely to be even more lasting in their performance and effect.

Objective Assessment of Success of Measures

Because of the increasing importance of atheroma in man's morbidity and mortality, means by which it may be surmounted present a serious challenge to the biological sciences. Before focusing on ways and means by which this challenge might be met, it will be instructive to stand back and consider how the ways and means are to be justified.

We still have no clear proof that the measures intended to halt or slow the progress of atheroma do in practice do so. The proof would depend on successful field trials which would be particularly difficult to plan because atheroma in different degrees affects the majority of people, it is slow in development, and difficult to grade in severity. This means that a worthwhile trial requires observation of a large number of people over a long time. Evidence of atherosclerosis would depend on such serious events as myocardial infarcts, cerebral thromboses, or limb amputations. An additional difficulty in such a field trial would be that the measure designed to diminish atheroma entail alteration of life time habits of diet and exercise, and it would be very difficult to ensure that these measures were being carried out because most people would revert to their previous way of life without realizing it.

Recognition of the difficulties should not deter attempts to make this advance. The comments of Fredrickson on field trials are relevant. "Field trials are indispensable. They will continue to be an ordeal. They lack glamour, they strain our resources and patience, and they protract the moment of truth to excruciating limits. Still, they are among the most challenging tests of our skills. I have no doubt that when the problem is well chosen, the study is appropriately designed, and that when all the populations concerned are made aware of the route and goal, the reward can be commensurate with the effort. If, in major medical dilemmas, the alternative is to pay the cost of perpetual uncertainty, have we really any choice?"

With realization of why it is difficult to produce incontestable evidence of the value of measures to prevent or slow the progress of atherosclerosis we have to learn what we can from individual experience. Some will claim that reduction of hyperlipidemia is a life-saving measure, others, more skeptical, will comment that disappearance of cholesterol from the bloodstream means that it has been deposited on the arterial wall. Our own experience, without controls, has been that some patients who have followed dietary and pharmaceutical advice to effect a reduction in the level of hyperlipidemia have experienced a halting of the progress of symptoms of arterial disease. Zelis and his colleagues observed three patients with type III hyperlipidemia and intermittent claudication. Following treatment with diet restriction (600 calories per diem for 25 days) and combined drug treatment (Clofibrate *) for 120 days, the symptom of intermittent claudication disappeared in one patient and diminished in the other two, and in all there was an increase in the maximum blood flow to the calf.

PRACTICAL CONSIDERATIONS

Symptoms

The symptoms of atherosclerosis are those of arterial obstruction which are dealt with in detail in Chapter 2. Intermittent claudication is the usual presenting symptom. Persistent foot pain, with or without ulceration is an advanced manifestation.

Signs

The outstanding sign of atherosclerosis in the limbs is loss or diminution of pulses. A common mistake is to assume that because aortoiliac disease has resulted in diminution of femoral pulses and loss of popliteals that the pedal pulses will also be absent; very often the collateral circulation round the high block is so good that peripheral pulses persist. Ischemia of the feet is unusual in the Leriche syndrome and when present is likely to be due to emboli.

Presence of good femoral pulses, weak or absent popliteal pulses with absent distal pulses and peripheral ischemia is suggestive of diabetic atherosclerosis. Some wasting of the limb muscles occurs with restriction of arterial supply, but unless this is unilateral it is unlikely to be a helpful clinical sign.

Treatment for Ambulant Patients

The following account is chiefly directed to the treatment of atherosclerosis of the limbs, though the general principles involved are to be followed in all types of vascular disease. If a

* Trademark, Ayerst Laboratorie.

patient cooperates with a doctor who follows the principles of good management, his life can be made happier and his limbs saved from amputation. Abstention from cigarette smoking is desirable in all arterial diseases, and imperative in thromboangiitis obliterans.

Foot Care for Poor Arterial Circulation

WALKING PATIENTS

1. *Keep warm.* Warmth relaxes the blood vessels and improves the circulation. Wear warm clothes during the day and keep your feet from getting chilled by using warm foot coverings: fleece lined boots and soft woolen socks for outside wear, woolen bootees and warm bedroom slippers for in the house. Keep as warm as possible in bed. You may find an electric blanket helpful. Wear soft knitted bed socks.

2. *Never* apply heat directly to your feet, nor allow anyone else to do so. Direct heat may burn them. Do not put your feet on a heating pad or hot water bottle, soak them in hot water, or expose them to the heat of a radiator, or to sunburn.

3. Protect your feet from injury. Never walk barefooted even in your bedroom, use warm bedroom slippers or bootees which cover and protect your feet from knocks. Wear soft, wide, round toed, well fitting shoes or boots in the house and outside, have them checked for fit by your podiatrist or doctor. The slightest injury to the skin of your feet should be reported to your doctor. Don't use adhesive, corn pads, or other medicated applications without consulting him.

4. Wash your feet daily with warm water and soap. Dry gently and thoroughly, especially between the toes, with a clean towel. If the skin is dry apply lanolin or a baby oil, if the skin is damp use foot powder.

5. Don't smoke.

6. Do not sit for long periods with your feet down, if you do fluid collects in them, makes them swell, and slows down healing. Never let anyone make you lie with your legs higher than your chest.

7. Have your feet treated by a skilled podiatrist. Be sure that he is aware of your poor circulation.

DISABLED PATIENTS (For the nurse)

1. See that your patient understands the instructions on foot care for walking patients (above).

2. The forces of gravity can help or hinder your patient's circulation. Your patient is likely to find this out for himself and may prefer sitting in a chair to lying in bed. When the feet are down in this position the blood reaches the toes but its return by the veins is hampered and edema develops. If you elevate his feet to disperse the edema you will endanger the circulation. You will make the best use of gravity if you have the head of the patients bed lifted on 6 to 9 inch wooden blocks.

3. In cases of severe ischemia the foot is easily damaged by rubbing or pressure:

a. Lift the weight of the bed clothes off the feet by using a cage or, failing that, by placing a pillow on the bottom sheet at the foot of the bed.

b. Pressure sores can develop on the foot, usually the heel. If the heels are pressing on the bottom sheet they can be kept lifted off by making a legging for the calf or calves by wrapping with plastic foam sheet. This should be no thicker than is required just to lift the foot clear of the bottom sheet, otherwise you are elevating the feet.

c. Wash any redness, blistering of the skin, or break in it with soap or pHisohex, and cover with sterile gauze. Inform the doctor.

When evidence of vascular impairment is found, it is important to exclude the possibility of a primary disease which may be accelerating the development of atherosclerosis. Diabetes mellitus, hypertension, hypothyroidism, hyperlipidemia, and polycythemia vera must be considered and treated if found. Of these it is relevant to consider the control of hyperlipidemia in more detail.

Diet remains the most important factor in the control of hyperlipidemia. For many years the main effort was in restriction of saturated fats. Then attention was directed to the salutory effects of ensuring that carbohydrate in the diet was in the form of starches rather than of sugars and limiting the intake to 120 to

150 grams per day. Most recent opinions are veering to the simple view that limitation of the caloric value is the most important advice in devising a diet. It is fortunate that type V is rarely encountered, for correction of the chylomicronemia requires restriction of fat, that of pro-β-lipoproteinemia restriction of carbohydrate, and the resulting high protein diet is expensive and difficult to maintain. On any diet alcohol should be restricted to reduce the hypertriglyceridemia. The following list gives ground rules for diet for patients with peripheral atheromatous disease.

Diet for Arterial Disease

DO NOT EAT:

1. Sugars of any kind including syrups, honey, fruit juices
2. Sugar-containing foods: cakes, pies, pastries
3. Milk, butter, cheeses and cream
4. Alcohol

SELECT DIET FROM:

1. Meats: chicken, bacon, beef, lamb, pork
2. Vegetables: except beets and parsnips
3. Starches (potatoes): one serving only. Use leafy vegetables.
4. Not more than one egg daily
5. Salad oils and salads
6. Use sugar substitutes—saccharine, etc., if required
7. Dietetic sodas
8. Not more than four slices of bread
9. A small amount of skimmed milk may be used on cereals
10. Nuts in moderation
11. Oleomargarine—no coconut, no milk

In addition to dietary control, various pharmaceutical preparations have been introduced to reduce hyperlipidemia. Clofibrate is used to reduce the levels of abnormal β-lipoproteins and pre-β-lipoproteins in patients with types III and IV when dietetic treatment has not been entirely successful. The combination of cholestyramine resin with a low cholesterol diet has been found to reduce the β-lipoprotein levels to, or near to, normal in familial Type II hyperlipoproteinemia. However, cholestyramine should be used with caution until more is known of its long term effects. Perhaps its use should be restricted to young patients with high β-lipoprotein levels when there is a family history of premature vascular disease. Cholestyramine may bind drugs and interfere with the absorption, so it should be given more than half an hour after their administration. Particular care is needed when it is given with oral anticoagulant drugs. Other drugs which have been recommended in the treatment of atherosclerosis are thyroxine, nicotinic acid and progestational analogues.

The patient with intermittent claudication should be encouraged to accept his disability and walk until pain stops him. If this advice is followed the physical effect is to promote the development of collateral circulation, the psychological effect, to encourage the patient to be more philosophical about his disability.

The patient with arteriosclerosis obliterans should choose his podiatrist as carefully as he chooses his surgeon. A good podiatrist will advise well fitting, warm and comfortable shoes, and give regular attention to his feet and toenails, thus providing prophylactic care. It is important that the podiatrist should be familiar with the effects of vascular disease.

In theory, vasodilator drugs are of doubtful value. Papaverine serves as an example of the paradox of the general dilator drug. This drug has the property of dilating arterial and arteriolar walls, but since its action is a general one when it is given intravenously in an effective dose, all arteries of the bodies are dilated, the blood pressure falls, and the blood flow distal to an obstruction is diminished rather than increased. However, if it is given by arterial infusion upstream of an obstructed artery, some increase in blood flow distally may be expected. One may imagine that if a drug has the property of dilating the arterioles of voluntary muscle it will do so on such arterioles throughout the body, whether or not there is an arterial obstruction. The result is that comparatively more blood will be directed to muscles with normal circulation, but it is doubtful whether the blood flow to those with arterial obstruction will be increased. Coffman and Mannick carried out a critical trial of the effects of vasodilator agents on symptoms and blood flow to the limbs both at rest and on exercise. The agents used were Rx Nylidrin, Isoxsuprine, tolazoline and nicotinyl alcohol. No evidence of improvement of symptoms or increase in blood flow to skin or to muscle on exercise was obtained. In spite of these theoretical objections, it is sometimes found that the prescription of a "vasodilating drug" may be of psychological value to the patient, and maybe to his doctor also. Isoxsuprine hydrochloride may help intermittent claudication and tolazoline hydrochloride, those with digital ischemia.

Treatment (Bed Patients)

When nocturnal pain disturbs his sleep the patient often takes to sleeping in a chair and develops dependent edema in his feet. This state can be avoided if analgesics and sedatives are supplied and the patient blocks up the head of his bed by 12 to 16 inches in order to increase the hydrostatic perfusion pressure to his feet. The legs of a patient with ischemic disease must *never* be raised above heart level, even to disperse edema.

Promotion of vasodilatation by heat is a complicated problem. Direct heat, by hot water bottles or heating pads, accelerates tissue metabolism, but an increase in blood flow cannot occur to supply the increased metabolism and to disperse the local overheating of the tissues. On the other hand, if the patient and his feet remain cold and vasoconstricted he loses the benefit of the vasodilatation afforded by warmth. A useful compromise is to get the patient to keep his body as warm as he can tolerate, even if this requires a heating cradle and heating pads for bed patients. His legs should be kept warm with bed socks and blankets. An unheated cradle over the feet helps to prevent trauma.

The patient with peripheral vascular disease is particularly liable to develop pressure sores or ulcers. This is because relatively light pressure on the tissues, such as the weight of the heel on the bed is more than the lowered peripheral arterial pressure, and ischemia of the tissue results from it. Pressure lesions are to be prevented by frequent change of position of the patient, and nursing him on foam, or preferably sheepskin bed overlays. A useful device to prevent pressure on the heels is to wrap the calf in a foam legging, just thick enough to clear the heels from resting on the bed.

When ulcers develop on ischemic feet, only bland local applications should be applied. Dry dressing alternated with wet saline or boric acid solutions or potassium permanganate in weak solution may be used as brief soaks once a day. Antibiotics are seldom required, for the cause of the lesion is not infection but ischemia, and the bacterial flora is usually a mixed one.

Surgical Treatment

At an early stage the possibility of arterial surgery to relieve the obstruction must be considered and arteriography carried out if necessary. The risk of arteriography is small, and the benefits may be great.

Aortoiliac disease may be treated surgically either by endarterectomy with extensive clearing out of the atheromatous material from the lower aorta and the iliac arteries, or synthetic grafts in place of the vessels. In occasional cases it may be undesirable to approach the aortoiliac region directly, either because the arterial disease is so extensive that it is unlikely that a graft can be inserted satisfactorily or because it is thought unwise to subject the patient to an intra-abdominal operation; under these circumstances an axillary-femoral graft has been shown to be feasible and effective. The results of the aortoiliac surgery are usually good, and patency of the vessels usually persists for long periods. Operative mortality is minimal and morbidity small. One possible surgical complication is the dislodgement of atheromatous material to form emboli in the leg (Fig. 2-2).

Though the patient's complaint of claudication is usually greatly, if not completely relieved, his complaint of sexual disability, which is often the chief reason for seeking help, is less likely to be relieved. May et al. examined this problem in 43 men who had had aortoiliac reconstructions for occlusive disease, one half of whom had had impairment of erection before operation. Seven were improved after the operation, but seven whose function had been normal before had impaired function afterwards. Sexual function seemed more likely to be impaired if it was necessary to extend the resection beyond the common iliac arteries. One possibility is that the pudendal arteries, narrowed by arteriosclerosis, may have the perfusion pressure within them further diminished by the bypass or by kinking of the artery so that impairment of erection results. Another cause for interference with sexual function is resection of the superior hypogastric sympathetic plexus (presacral nerve) during aortoiliac surgery. When this occurs the ability to ejaculate is liable to be lost, as after lumbar sympathectomy, which is described below. Sabri and Cotton have described how this complication can be mostly avoided. At the operation the right superior hypogastric plexus is sacrificed but the left is carefully preserved by burrowing under the vascular pedicle supplying the rectum and mobilizing the left common iliac artery and its bifurcation to the left of the sigmoid colon. By this means the left superior hypogastric plexus is preserved, and the fibers from the lumbar chain to it remain intact. With these precautions the man who was impotent before the operation because atheroma of the aortoiliac region had resulted in reduced perfusion pressure in the pudendal arteries may have his potency restored, and the others may be protected from impotency.

Femoropopliteal reconstruction has become commonplace in vascular surgery with a choice of operation between endarterectomy or insertion of an aterial bypass. The range of endarterectomy is from a closed method in which successive catheters each of greater diameter are pushed as bougies down the artery, to an open method in which the whole length of the artery is opened up, the occluding substance scooped out and the artery closed by means of a long strip of vein which forms a gusset. Usually, however, endarterectomy is used only when the stenosis is localized to a short segment. Early experience with femoropopliteal bypass procedures showed that a bypass of autogenous vein remained patent for much longer periods than any other material so that synthetic grafts are used below the inguinal ligament only when there is no alternative. Use of autogenous vein grafts limits the surgeon to such veins as are available and calls into play technical ingenuity to make a contracted saphenous vein bridge the arterial gap and provide wide strong anastomoses at the two openings into the artery. Venous grafts left in situ with destruction of the valves have been used as long bypass grafts; the technique requires a full length incision over the vein, meticulous removal of the valves to avoid thrombosis, and an equally meticulous tying off of branches which might otherwise form arteriovenous fistulae. The use of venous homografts needs to be more fully explored.

Tibial and peroneal arteries are often severely affected in patients over 70 years of age and much earlier than that if the patient is diabetic. In these cases a femoropopliteal bypass may be technically feasible, but if the "run-off" is insufficient, the slow flow of blood in the reconstructed artery is liable to thrombosis. In recent years surgical progress has made it possible to extend venous grafts into the tibial and peroneal arteries with encouraging results.

The effects of sympathectomy on the circulation to the limbs is described in Chapter 1 and may be summarized as a transient (10 days) increase in blood flow to the whole limb, after which blood flow to the hands and feet remains increased but the blood flow to the proximal parts of the limb reverts to normal levels. The increase of blood flow in the hands persists for about a year but lasts considerably longer in the feet. The failure of sympathectomy to maintain a lasting increase in blood flow to more proximal parts of the limb may explain its failure to relieve the symptom of intermittent claudication. When arterial disease is mostly in the feet and lower calves, as in thromboangiitis obliterans, sympathectomy has often been of value in healing cutaneous lesions. Sympathectomy often relieves the pain of causalgia (see p. 196) and so may relieve such pain as may be caused by a similar mechanism in chronic ischemia; however, the evidence for this is very doubtful. At times when arterial disease is so extensive that no reconstructive surgery seems possible but when the patient is threatened with loss of a limb there is a tendency to "see what sympathectomy can do." This tendency should be resisted. Sympathectomy cannot be expected to open up thrombosed arteries, and beneficial results almost never follow the operation when done for such purposes. Nor should it be overlooked that the morbidity of an abdominal operation increases in older and more feeble patients.

One untoward effect of sympathectomy which should be explained to the patient before operation is the phenomenon of postsympathectomy neuralgia. This is a neuralgic pain in the shoulder and deltoid region following cervicodorsal sympathectomy and in the buttocks and thigh following lumbar sympathectomy. The onset of this pain tends to be about 10 days after the surgery so that by the time it arises the patient is about to leave the hospital and does not wish to delay his departure because of a new complaint, with the result that the hospital based surgeons tend to overlook this complication of the operation. More than one third of postsympathectomy patients experience such neuralgia, and in some the discomfort is severe. The pain responds fairly well to analgesics, but an important fact to convey to the patient is that many suffer this complication after sympathectomy, and it always abates within 3 or 4 months, and sometimes long before that.

Another complication of sympathectomy is interference with sexual function, in males, that is, for the effect on sexual function of females does not appear to have been recorded. Most of the reports on this question are less precise than might be wished. One reason is that sexual function is sensitive to psychological influences and another is that aortoiliac disease itself may cause impotence and may either be relieved or made worse by the operation.

Early reports on diminution of sexual function following sympathectomy were concerned with interference with penile erection after the operation. This complication appeared to be due to severance of the nervi erigentes from central stimulation, and it was found that the path was less frequently interrupted if the first lumbar sympathetic ganglia were left intact. Even if the first ganglia are left intact another form of impotence may arise following bilateral lumbar sympathectomy, that is interference with the ability to ejaculate (dry orgasm). This symptom has also been noticed to follow resection of the presacral plexus of sympathetic nerves during reconstruction of the terminal aorta.

Intractable pain and extending ulcers of the feet are serious results of arterial disease. For the relief of pain percutaneous cordotomy has been tried, and in most cases is effective in interrupting the pain, but much is still to be learned about the selection of suitable cases. Intractable pain may eventually require that the limb, or a portion of it, be amputated. The loss of a limb is a serious physical and psychological blow to an elderly patient, and with few exceptions the expectation of life is greatly reduced when the need for it arises. It is a mistake to attempt to coerce a reluctant patient into amputation, but when the need arises the patient should be gently and firmly made aware of the situation. The operation should be carried out promptly when the patient agrees to it.

Following surgery a careful check should be kept on the distal pulses and reexploration of the affected vessel carried out promptly if there is reason to believe that thrombosis has occurred in it. Postoperative anticoagulation does not materially reduce the threat of arterial thrombosis but may lead to hematoma formation in the operative site.

Edema of the operated limb frequently occurs. This may be due to hyperemia, or to venous obstruction by extravasation. Venous thrombosis, however, may be the cause when the benefits of anticoagulation therapy must be balanced against the drawbacks. To reduce the chance of venous thrombosis the patient should be mobilized as soon as feasible after the operation.

Patients who have had prolonged and severe ischemia of the foot may complain of a causalgia-like pain in it when circulation has been restored. This usually responds to reassurance and analgesics.

REFERENCES

Distribution of Atherosclerosis

Lindbom, A.: Arteriosclerosis and arterial thrombosis in the lower limb. A roentgenological study. Acta Radiol. [Suppl.], *80*:1, 1950.

Mitchell, J.R.A. and Schwartz, C.J.: Arterial Disease. Philadelphia, F.A. Davis, 1965.

Hypertension and Atherosclerosis

Freis, Edward D.: Medical treatment of chronic hypertension. Modern Concepts of Cardiovascular Disease, *40*:17, 1971.

Roberts, J.C., Moses, C. and Wilkins, R.W.: Autopsy studies in atherosclerosis. Circulation, *20*:511, 1959.

Hyperlipoproteinemia and Atherosclerosis

Fredrickson, D.S., Levy, R.I., and Lees, R.S.: Fat transport in lipoproteins—an integrated approach to mechanisms and disorders. New Eng. J. Med., *276*: 32, 94, 148, 215, 273; 1967.

Greenhalgh, R.M., Lewis, B., Rosengarten, D.S., Calnan, J.S., Mervart, I. and Martin, P.: Serum lipids and lipoproteins in peripheral vascular disease. Lancet, *2*:947, 1971.

Kuo, P.R.: Atherosclerosis in Man; Genetic and Metabolic Implications of Hyperlipidemia. *In* Conn, H.L. and Horwitz, O. (eds.): Cardiac and Vascular Diseases. Philadelphia, Lea & Febiger, 1971.

Stack, J.: Risks of ischaemic heart disease in familial hyperlipoproteinaemic states. Lancet, *2*:1380, 1969.

Hyperglycemia and Atherosclerosis

Friedman, S.A., Holling, H.E. and Roberts, B.: Etiological factors in aortoiliac and femoropopliteal vascular disease (the Leriche syndrome). New Eng. J. Med., *271*:1382, 1964.

Gensler, S.W., et al.: Study of vascular lesions in diabetic and non-diabetic patients. Arch. Surg., *91*:617, 1965.

Strandness, D.E., Jr., Priest, R.E. and Gibbons, G.E.: A combined clinical and pathological study of diabetic and non-diabetic peripheral arterial disease. Diabetes, *13*:366, 1964.

Exercise and Atherosclerosis

Kannel, B.: Habitual level of physical activity and risk of coronary heart disease: The Framingham study. Canad. Med. Asso. J., *96*:811, 1967.

Field Trials

Fredrickson, D.S.: The field trial. Bull. N.Y. Acad. Med., *44*:985, 1968.

Effect of Treatment

Coffman, J.D. and Mannick, J.A.: Failure of vasodilator drugs in arteriosclerosis obliterans. Ann. Int. Med., *76*:35, 1972.

Zelis, R., Mason, D.T., Braunwald, E. and Levy, R.I.: Effects of hyperlipiproteinemias and their treatment on the peripheral J. Clin. Invest. Circulation. J.S.I., *49*:1007, 1970.

Surgical Treatment

May, A.G., DeWeese, J.A., Rob, C.F.: Changes in sexual function following operation on the abdominal aorta. Surgery, *65*:41, 1969.

Sabri, S. and Cotton, L.T.: Sexual function following aortoiliac reconstruction. Lancet, *2*:1218, 1971.

5

Medial Arteriosclerosis
and Aneurysms

Medial arteriosclerosis is the most common cause of aneurysms at the present time. The medial coat of the aorta and major arteries fragments, resulting in weakening and lessened resilience of the arterial wall so that it is likely to be stretched by the force of arterial pressure. Medial arteriosclerosis affects all major arteries, but its effects are seen most frequently in the abdominal aorta, less frequently in the iliac, popliteal arteries and in the femoral artery distal to the inguinal ligament, and rarely in the carotid arteries. When the wall is weakened the whole vessel is liable to be dilated, but if the vessel wall is weaker over one

TABLE 5-1. DISTINCTION BETWEEN ATHEROSCLEROSIS OBLITERANS AND MEDIAL ARTERIOSCLEROSIS

	ATHEROSCLEROSIS OBLITERANS	MEDIAL ARTERIOSCLEROSIS
Age Incidence	Over 45 years	Over 60 years
Sex Preponderance	Male and post meno-pausal female	Male predominantly
Location in Arterial System	Aorto-femoral, coronary, cerebral	Aorto-femoral
Early Histological Changes	Deposition of atheroma on intima	Fragmentation of elastica of media
Effect on Arterial Lumen	Narrowing	Dilatation
Progress Accelerated by	Hypertension, diabetes, hyperlipidemia	Hypertension
Increase in Mortality * from 1942 to 1962	64%	400%

* Based on figures from the Registrar General of England Wales' Report.

91

area or if for some reason there is a local increase in distending pressure, that portion of the vessel is liable to blow out and form an aneurysm.

The name medial arteriosclerosis is likely to confuse, but less so than the commonly used term arteriosclerotic aneurysm. The latter term confuses the condition with that of atherosclerosis. The distinction is made clear in Table 5-1. Arteriosclerosis is an unsuitable word to use, for it describes a weakened wall as a hardened one. Arteriectasia has been used to describe the dilated condition of the vessel affected by medial arteriosclerosis, but though it is a good descriptive term, it has not come into general use.

ETIOLOGY

Medial arteriosclerosis is associated with advancing age and is probably constitutional. When Osler wrote on the subject of abdominal aneurysm in 1905, four of his cases were judged to be nonsyphilitic (average age 54), whereas 12 were syphilitic (average age 39 years). Since that time syphilis has been virtually eliminated as a cause of abdominal aneurysm, and old age has taken its place.

The question of why aneurysms form in certain locations more frequently than others is an interesting topic for theorizing. A patient with medial arteriosclerosis is likely to be hypertensive, and the manifestations of his disease are found in the lower half of the body where the hydrostatic forces resulting from the upright posture reinforce the stress of the arterial pressure. An aneurysm is liable to occur in a segment of the vessel which is not fixed in position by major branches and where the resistance to expansion of the surrounding tissues is small. In accounting for the site of development of an aneurysm Malcolm has proposed that pulse waves and their reflections resonate in the arterial system forming nodes and antinodes. Major branches arise at a node, as at the level of the renal arteries, and there atheromatous stenosis is liable to occur. Between the renal arteries and the bifurcation of the aorta there is only one major branch. Over this section an antinode develops, and it is here that an aneurysm is liable to occur. A simpler theory is that the tissues around the abdominal aorta, in the femoral triangle, and at the distal end of Hunter's canal, offer less resistance to its aneurysmal expansion. The rarity of aneurysms of this type in the carotid artery may be accounted for by the lower arterial pressure in it than in the lower part of the body when the patient is standing upright.

INCIDENCE

Over the past 20 years there has been a remarkable rate of increase in the incidence of nonsyphilitic aneurysm compared to the more familiar rate of increase of atherosclerosis in the population (See Tables 5-1 and 5-2). Much of this rate of increase

TABLE 5-2. MORTALITY FIGURES *

	1942	1962	% INCREASE
Arteriosclerotic Heart Disease	96,953	150,621	57
Cerebro-Thromboembolism	16,143	37,872	112
Diseases of Arteries	11,778	15,508	31
Summation	124,874	204,001	64
Aneurysm (nonsyphilitic)	586	3,042	419

* These figures are derived from those given by Eastcott from the mortality reports of the Registrar General of England and Wales.

may be attributed to a longer life span of the population, and some to an increase in the diagnosis of abdominal aneurysm since it has become possible to treat it surgically. The age of the patients we have studied personally is given by the figures published by Brooke Roberts and his surgical colleagues. Of 390 patients selected for resection of an abdominal aneurysm, 346 were men and 44 were women. The ages of the patients ranged from 31 to 79 years with a mean age of 64. The preponderance of males with this condition is clear, but the reason for it is not known. Since the group is one selected for surgical treatment, older patients would be excluded, and therefore it appears that the average patient with aortic aneurysm is a man in his late sixties.

ABDOMINAL ANEURYSM

Symptoms

Even a large aneurysm may give rise to no symptoms, the patient being aware of a large pulsating mass in his abdomen, but with no other complaints. Aches and pains are a concomitant of advancing age so that many of the symptoms which are attributed to aneurysm may not in fact be due to that cause. We have, however, been impressed by the number of patients with persistent low back pain who lost the symptom after their aneurysm had been resected. The relative painlessness of many aneurysms today contrasts with Osler's experience: "pain of a persistent, often of an agonizing character was present in 13 of the 16 cases. It is usually the first indication of trouble, and throughout remains the feature, reaching an intensity not met with in any other disease." The contrast between the painlessness of present day abdominal aneurysms and the painfulness of those seen at the beginning of the century may well be due to the difference between an aneurysm due to syphilis, and one due to medial arteriosclerosis, for the syphilitic aneurysm has more invasive properties as is seen by erosion of the lumbar vertebrae in this condition.

When symptoms arise from an abdominal aneurysm there is a real danger that the aneurysm is about to rupture, is leaking, or has ruptured. A useful maxim for the physician is that the onset of definite symptoms in a patient with abdominal aneurysm is due to rupture until proved otherwise. It is wise to get the patient to the surgeon, for delay is dangerous and the mortality rate for ruptured aneurysm is high. Rupture into the abdominal cavity is likely to be fatal so quickly that it is seldom that the patient lives long enough to be seen by a physician. If rupture occurs into the retroperitoneal space, the bleeding is contained so that for some hours the patient may remain fit enough to be transferred for surgery. During this interim the physician needs to act decisively and promptly. The aneurysm may not be palpable because of diminished pressure in it and increased tone of the muscles of the abdominal wall covering it, but out in either flank may be found a tender swelling which is sometimes mistaken for an abscess unless the definite pulsation within it is detected. Supportive findings are a fall of blood pressure and of hemoglobin. but action should not wait until these are available. The pain of a slowly leaking aneurysm may suggest diverticulosis, or renal colic if the pain strikes down into the testicles. If oozing occurs into the bowel melena may be a presenting feature.

Signs

Physical examination of men over 55 years should always pay special attention to the possibility of an abdominal aneurysm. Pointers towards presence of medial arteriosclerosis are: a high systolic pressure with a widened pulse pressure, femoral arteries of unduly wide caliber, or popliteal pulsation which is unusually easily felt. Unusual abdominal pulsation is often appreciated by inspection of the abdomen. Epigastric pulsation in slender persons is not unusual. In slender females pulsation felt here can be considered normal. Osler quotes Allan Burns on this point: "I suppose there is no young physician who has not diagnosed as aneurysm of the aorta the preternatural pulsation of the vessel. In any suspected case it is well to be skeptical, particularly in women, in whom aneurysm is excessively rare."

An epigastric tumor with pulsation in either man or woman raises the question of whether the tumor is an aneurysm or whether it is a pancreatic cyst or pseudo-cyst through which aortic pulsation is being transmitted. Unless the pulsation in the epigastrium is definitely expansible the condition is more likely to be pulsation transmitted through a pancreatic tumor. Pulsation felt in a male abdomen above and to the left of the umbilicus and below and to the right is very suggestive of abdominal aneurysm.

The diagnosis is certain when the outlines of an expansile pulsatile mass can be felt, but in many cases the clinical diagnosis is not certain. Palpation should always be gentle. It is good practice to listen for bruits, though the murmurs associated with abdominal aneurysms have no particular significance, unless they give rise to the suspicion of an A-V fistula.

Investigations

When physical examination indicates that an abdominal aneurysm is present, it is wise to pause and decide whether the patient is a suitable candidate for excision and replacement. If at this stage the decision is against elective surgery, there is no point in going on into further diagnostic studies, and only in exceptional circumstances need the patient be told of the possibility of the aneurysm, though his younger relatives should be warned of it and the need for prompt action should the patient develop unusual abdominal pain or bleeding.

If surgical treatment is a possibility, the next diagnostic step is a flat plate of the abdomen, in particular a lateral film. Calcium in the wall of the aneurysm or in the layers of the thrombus within it often will outline the vessel and show its dilatation. In preparation for surgery it has been the practice to carry out aortography "to see whether the aneurysm involves the renal arteries" though it seldom does. In favor of an aortogram is that it (a) can usefully confirm or deny a provisional diagnosis of aneurysm; (b) can indicate whether the effects of medial arteriosclerosis have extended into the iliac and femoral arteries, or whether there are other unsuspected aneurysms; (c) may rarely show other abnormalities such as a horsehoe kidney or accessory renal arteries; (d) may demonstrate thrombus within the aneurysmal sac, and thrombotic emboli in the distal vessels; and (e) can show the anastomoses between the inferior mesenteric artery and the superior and hypogastric arteries and so give useful information whether the inferior mesenteric artery can be sacrificed at operation.

Aortography, however, is a fallible investigation. If the aneurysm contains much thrombus, the dilatation of the vessel may not be shown. In other cases anterior-posterior bends in the artery may give a false impression that the aneurysm involves the renal arteries when in fact it does not. It is questionable whether an aortogram is required in all cases because the renal arteries are seldom involved in the aneurysm and advances in surgical technique have made it possible to cope with this situation if they are. In all cases consideration should be given to the possibility that a "venous" aortogram could give the information required of an "arterial" aortogram. Injection of the dye into a vein gives less definition than when it is injected directly into the aorta, but the procedure is less protracted and attended by fewer complications.

Surgical Management

Before a physician comes to a decision whether or not to refer his patient for surgical treatment of an aortic aneurysm he should be very sure that an aneurysm is present. The dividing line here is an arbitrary one. If the aorta of a slim female measures 3.5 cm. in diameter it is significantly dilated; but an aorta of this diameter in a large male could be within normal limits. Once an aorta has expanded it is likely to continue to expand. One reason for this is the physical one described by LaPlace's law, that is, as the radius of a tube increases the tension within the wall increases in proportion. Another reason for expansion is a pathological one that as the aortic wall is thinned it is replaced by less resilient fibrous tissue. We may expect that all aortic aneurysms would enlarge rapidly towards rupture, but experience teaches that their course shows great variability. Some aneurysms enlarge and progress towards rupture within a few months, whereas others are slow to enlarge and remain asymptomatic for years. Reasons for this variability are hard to determine.

One having decided that an aneurysm is present we might consider the case for conservative treatment. Because medial arteriosclerosis occurs with advancing age it is also associated with an increased incidence of cancer and coronary and cerebral vascular disease. The associated diseases are equally likely to cause death. The question to be asked therefore is whether the benefit of surgical treatment is sufficient to justify advising it for a patient whose aneurysm gives rise to no symptoms and who is just as likely to succumb to another disease. All published figures indicate that more patients will survive longer if they have had the benefit of surgery, but it is difficult to match surgical and non-surgical groups for a true comparison. Szilagyi (1966) reported on a group of 223 patients with abdominal aneurysm treated from 1944 through 1965 without surgery, for comparison with a similar group treated with resection of the aneurysm. Best results were obtained in patients having an aneurysm less than 6 cm. in diameter: 47 per cent survived 5 years without operation but 67 per cent of those who had operations survived 5 years. However, the two groups were not altogether comparable for those treated nonsurgically were observed in the earlier years and those treated surgically in the later years. This fact affects results, since it was during this period that improvements in both medical and surgical management occurred.

In 1927, before surgery of the aorta was feasible, Colt estimated that the average duration of life from the first onset of symptoms was 18 to 24 months. In 1950, about the time that aortic surgery was beginning to be carried out, Estes found that 7 of 37 patients with abdominal aneurysm survived 5 years. In 1962 Schatz et al. reported that 12 of 33 patients survived 5 years, and in 1967 Steinberg and Tobier found that half the patients not treated with surgery survived 6 years. The different conditions of the patients at the time of diagnosis and the different causes of death make these figures informative only in the broadest sense. They suggest that the expectation of life after an aneurysm has been diagnosed has increased during the last 40 years, even in the absence of surgical treatment. The reason for this improvement may well be largely the effectiveness of antihypertensive treatment, but other reasons contribute. Earlier records included a number of patients whose aneurysms were syphilitic; these may have had a worse prognosis. With the development of surgical treatment interest in the condition has resulted in earlier diagnosis. Advances of treatment of associated conditions, particularly pulmonary and urinary infections, have contributed to a more favorable prognosis.

If the expectation of life has increased for a patient with abdominal aneurysm treated without surgery, it has increased even more if his aneurysm can be resected, for then the advances in medical and surgical treatment of the last 20 years supplement each other. The most telling argument in favor of surgical treatment is the advances in technique and management which have resulted in a remarkable reduction in the operative mortality of abdominal aneurysms. Earlier figures for this mortality were around 12 per cent, but between May, 1967, and January, 1970, 96 patients had resection of an abdominal aneurysm at the Hospital of the University of Pennsylvania without a single operative death, a record that stands at the time of writing 2 years later. This is a strong reason for advocating surgical treatment, for without such treatment the fear of rupture of the aneurysm is ever present, and even with prompt surgical intervention the mortality for this condition remains high.

Strong reasons for advising prompt surgical treatment are: (1) an isolated lesion in a healthy person, (2) an enlarging aneurysm, or one more than 6 cm. in diameter, and (3) rupture or suspicion of impending rupture.

A reason for not pressing for surgical treatment would be a patient's decided reluctance for surgery. Other reasons for not advising surgical treatment are: (1) somatic, and/or psychic senile degeneration; (2) extensive medial arteriosclerosis affecting iliac and femoral arteries in addition to the aorta; (3) advanced pulmonary disease; (4) advanced coronary, cerebral, or peripheral arteriosclerosis; and (5) other malignant disease. Old age is not of itself a contraindication to advising surgery for aortic aneurysm, but most physicians would be reluctant to advise surgery after the age of 75. Cardiac disease and some degree of cerebrovascular involvement is often present and does not preclude a satisfactory result from operation, but in some cases these conditions are so severe that the risk of surgery is inadvisable.

In the series at the Hospital of the University of Pennsylvania patients with large aneurysms and aneurysms associated with widespread dilatation of the arterial system, or distal aneurysms and occlusions fared less well. Patients with peripheral vascular disease in addition to the aneurysm also had a less favorable prognosis. On the whole, patients with cardiac disease fared well, though clearly severe cardiac disease would weight a decision against surgery. Moderate cerebrovascular disease did not result in an increased risk of operation, but when the patient is suffering from transient ischemic attacks as a result of stenosis of the internal carotid artery the question arises whether the aorta or the carotid artery should be first dealt with. Usually it is wise to relieve the carotid stenosis before resecting the aneurysm because of the danger of reduction of carotid arterial pressure during surgery. Chronic obstructive pulmonary disease carries an additional hazard.

Nonsurgical Management

When surgical excision is not advisable the patient should be advised against undue muscular exertion. He must be instructed to seek medical treatment if he has unusual abdominal pain or evidence of melena. He should be examined at intervals of not more than 3 months, and a record should be made of the estimated size of his aneurysm. Hypertension must be effectively treated. In medical management of dissecting aneurysm it has been found that dampening of the systolic thrust of the arterial pulse by means of a β-blocker such as propanalol is useful, and it has been suggested that this form of treatment may be useful in the medical management of an aortic aneurysm. We have not used this form of long term therapy because of the danger of precipitating cardiac failure. Particular attention should be paid to the possibility of urinary obstruction and infection, and also pulmonary obstructive disease.

ILIAC AND FEMORAL ANEURYSMS

Medial arteriosclerosis affects the iliac and femoral arteries as it affects the aorta, and it is usual to find these arteries dilated when an aortic aneurysm is present. The iliac arteries may be affected before the aorta, in which case the diagnosis of iliac aneurysm may be missed. Femoral aneurysms are less likely to be missed since the vessel is easily palpable.

The aneurysms of these vessels are less dangerous to life than an aortic aneurysm for they are less likely to rupture, and the consequences are less serious if they do. Their threat is that of the formation of thrombus within them to obstruction of the lumen, or more likely to serve as a source of emboli. The preferred method of treatment is surgical unless the disease is too widespread.

POPLITEAL ANEURYSMS

Medial arteriosclerosis is the most frequent cause of popliteal aneurysm. For a number of reasons the lesion may exist unrecognized for years. Some physicians, early in their careers, decide that the palpation of popliteal pulses is beyond their capability, and since the patient is customarily examined only when he is lying on his back the obvious pulsation in the popliteal fossa may be missed. When aneurysms are large the patient will himself call attention to them (Fig. 5-1).

Patients may give a characteristic history or recurrent attacks of painful cyanosed areas on the toes of one leg which gradually regress, only to be followed by a fresh crop. The localized areas of ischemia contrast with the normal looking skin of the remainder of the foot (Fig. 2-2) and the condition in connection with a popliteal aneurysm is usually unilateral. Figure 5-2 shows an unusual effect of an embolus from a popliteal aneurysm which lodged in a cutaneous branch of the anterior tibial artery.

In the absence of symptoms, diagnosis depends on one's assessment of the width of the popliteal artery pulsation; aneurysm is to be considered when the pulsatile area is more than 1.5 cm. wide. When a nonpulsatile swelling is felt in the popliteal space other diagnoses must be considered, including that of a Baker's cyst.

Large aneurysms may cause pressure on the popliteal vein

PADDINGTON TECHNICAL
COLLEGE LIBRARY,
3, PADDINGTON GREEN,
LONDON, W.2.

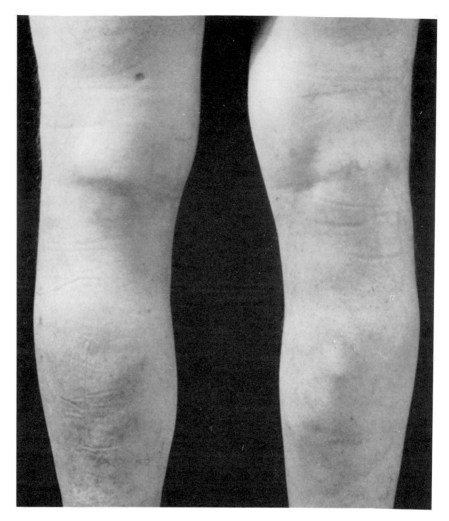

Fig. 5-1. Bilateral popliteal aneurysms. The left calf shows dilated cutaneous veins resulting from pressure of the aneurysm on the lesser saphenous vein.

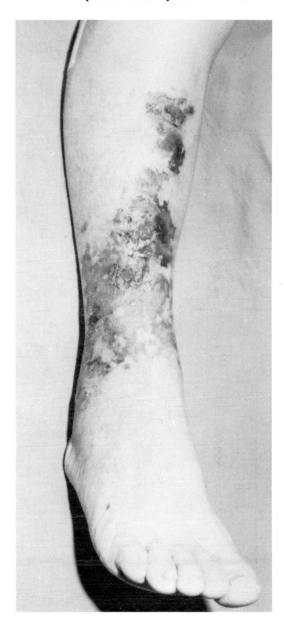

Fig. 5-2. Localized ischemia of the skin resulting from an embolus from a popliteal aneurysm.

resulting in venous obstruction and sometimes venous thrombosis. Likewise, pressure on the tibial nerve may result in a neurologic deficit. An arteriogram may fail to show the aneurysm which has been diagnosed from clinical examination, this is possibly because thrombus in the aneurysm has narrowed the lumen, however, even in these cases the radiologist may notice that the dye passes very slowly down the artery.

Not all popliteal aneurysms are due to medial arteriosclerosis. In the early 19th century popliteal aneurysms were called "post boy's aneurysm" and were considered to be syphilitic. The post boy was the man who rode crouched on the neck of one of the leading pair of horses of a post chaise. Presumably the combination of the flexed knee position whilst on duty, and the opportunities for promiscuity when off duty, resulted in the frequent occurrence of syphilitic popliteal aneurysms in these men. Perhaps this story has an element of myth, for syphilitic aneurysms of peripheral arteries seem to be very rare. The arteriogram shown in Figure 5-3 is the only popliteal aneurysm which I have seen to be associated with syphilis. The patient was not a post boy, but a veteran who had acquired syphilis during service in Southeast Asia during World War II.

An alternate cause of aneurysm in this young man might have been the popliteal entrapment syndrome. This is congenital and usually bilateral. The popliteal artery runs first over and then under the medial head of the gastrocnemius so that it passes medially to the tendinous insertion of the muscle and may be compressed and constricted by it against the medial femoral condyle. The usual presentation is of intermittent claudication in a young man with no apparent vascular disease. In the early stages an arteriogram shows medial displacement of the artery and perhaps stenosis at the level of the medial femoral condyle. If the condition remains unrecognized, poststenotic aneurysmal

Fig. 5-3. Popliteal aneurysm in a man of 36 who had acquired syphilis in Southeast Asia during World War II. The aneurysm was excised but no pathological report is available. Popliteal artery entrapment (see text) was a possible cause of the condition.

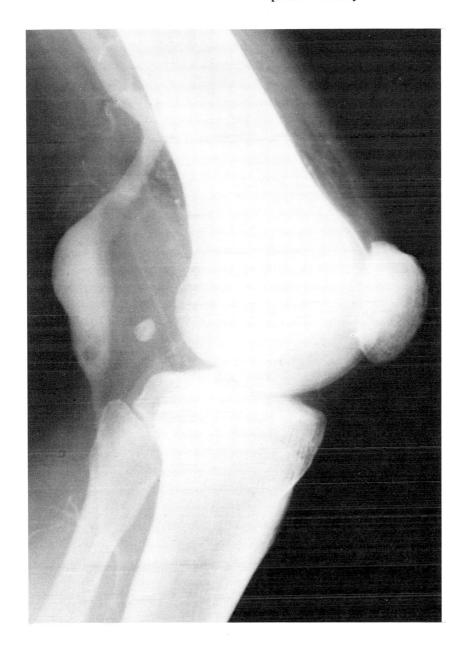

formation may occur. In the arteriogram shown, there is an acute bending of the artery which could have been due to medial displacement of the vessel by the medial head of the gastrocnemius, a filling defect representing the stenosis, and the fusiform appearance of an aneurysm due to post stenotic dilatation. The presumed point of compression, however, seems to be more proximal than is to be expected in the popliteal entrapment syndrome.

DISSECTING ANEURYSM

Dissecting aneurysm or hematoma is the result of extravasation of blood in the medial coats of the aorta which separates intima and adventitial layers. The tear in the intima through which the aortic blood pulses is usually in the ascending aorta. As the extravasation expands in the aortic wall major arterial branches are liable to be occluded, and because of this dissecting aneurysm is to be considered in the differential diagnosis of arterial obstruction.

The pathological process which facilitates dissection of the aorta is customarily said to be "arteriosclerosis." By this term it is inferred that atheromatous deposits on the intima of the aorta so weaken it as to render it liable to be torn, and that medial arteriosclerosis has so fragmented the muscular and elastic coats of the aorta as to make them more prone to disruption by the advancing hematoma.

The majority of patients with dissecting aneurysm are elderly and hypertensive, but the condition may occur in young patients in association with Marfan's syndrome, Erdheim's cystic medial necrosis, and occasionally with pregnancy. Trauma usually tears through the aortic wall instead of causing a dissection. Occasionally the condition may present as ischemia of one or both legs. In these cases a history of preceding chest pain is usually obtained, so both myocardial infarction with embolus and dissecting aneurysm extending to the iliac arteries are to be considered as causes for the ischemia.

Dissection is suggested by pain of sudden maximal onset, of a tearing quality and with a feeling of overwhelming distension or tightness. Often in dissection the chest pain abates in a few hours and moves down into the abdominal region. In dissection the peripheral ischemia is likely to occur within hours of the chest pain, whereas in myocardial infarction with embolus the interval between chest pain and ischemia is likely to be measured in days.

Early diagnosis depends largely on the history, for this is a lesion of symptoms rather than signs. The most important diagnostic measure is a chest radiograph in which the dissecting aneurysm shows as a widening of the superior mediastinum with hazy margins which later become clearer and sometimes lobulated. An aortogram with dye injected intraarterially or intravenously may be helpful. Electrocardiography should exclude myocardial infarction and this exclusion is important, for anticoagulant therapy in dissecting aneurysm is contraindicated.

Surgical treatment of dissecting aneurysm is attended by a distressing mortality, and medical treatment (with the hypotensive agents trimethaphan immediately and reserpine and guanethidine later) is preferred.

When dissection has involved the iliac artery so severely that its occlusion threatens the viability of the limb, a decision may be made to explore the artery as far as the aortic bifurcation with the object of restoring arterial flow. Even if such local surgical intervention is required, hypotensive rather than surgical treatment of the primary lesion of the aortic arch is still to be preferred.

REFERENCES

Hemodynamics of Aneurysm Formation

Malcolm, J.E..: Blood Pressure Sounds and Their Meanings. p. 84 et seq. London, Heiniman, 1957.

Age and Sex of Patients with Aneurysm of the Abdominal Aorta

Baker, A.G., Jr., Roberts, B., Berkowitz, H.D., and Barker, C.F.: Risk of excision of abdominal aortic aneurysms. Surgery, *68*:1129, 1970.

Osler, W.: Aneurysms of the abdominal aorta. Lancet, *2*:1089, 1905.

Increase in Deaths from Nonsyphilitic Aneurysm

Eastcott, H.H.G.: Arterial Surgery. p. 1. Philadelphia, J.B. Lippincott, 1969.

Survival of Patients After Diagnosis of Aneurysm

Colt, G.H.: The clinical duration of saccular aortic aneurysm in British born subjects. Quart. J. Med., *20*:331, 1927.

Estes, J.E.: Abdominal aortic aneurysm: a study of 102 cases. Circulation, *2*:258, 1950.

Schatz, I.J., Fairburn, J.F., and Juergens, J.L. Abdominal aortic aneurysms: a reappraisal. Circulation, *26*:200, 1962.

Steinberg, I., Tobier, N.: Study of 200 consecutive patients with abdominal aneurysms diagnosed by intravenous aortography. Comparative longevity with and without aneurysmectomy. Circulation, *35*:530, 1967.

Szilagyi, D.E., Smith, R.F., DeRusso, F.J., Elliot, J.P. and Sherrin, F.W.: Contribution of abdominal aortic aneurysmectomy to prolongation of life. Ann. Surg., *164*:678, 1966.

Treatment of Dissecting Aneurysm

Wheat, M.W., Palmer, R.F., Bartley, T.D. and Feelman, R.C.: Treatment of dissecting aneurysms of the aorta without surgery. Journal of Thoracic Cardiovascular Surgery, *50*:364, 1965.

6

Arteriovenous Fistula

HISTORY

A-V fistulae have proved of great interest both in clinical practice and in the experimental laboratory. Osler said of them that no lesion illustrates so well how borderless are the fields of medicine and science. It was William Hunter, in 1762, who first described how an aneurysm which was part of a fistulous connection between artery and vein differed from a simple aneurysm. This description was an important advance towards using Harvey's conception of the circulation in the explanation of disease states. Hunter's recognition that the bloodstream might pass directly from the high pressure artery to the low pressure vein and thereby bypass Harvey's "secret anastomoses" was conceived in terms of circulation of the blood and is thus an early, if not the first, application of the concept of circulation of blood to clinical medicine. Since that time experimental observations on A-V fistulae have contributed greatly to our understanding of the responses of the heart and circulation to the stress of a large leak of blood directly from the artery into the vein. Acquired A-V fistulae are usually the result of trauma. They are more frequently acquired in war time.

GENERAL EFFECTS

A-V fistulae, acquired or congenital, large or small, affect the circulation in a similar manner and to a degree dependent on the size of the fistula. A fistula may be considered as a thirsty mouth requiring ever more blood and steadily becoming larger and putting more strain on the local and general circulation.

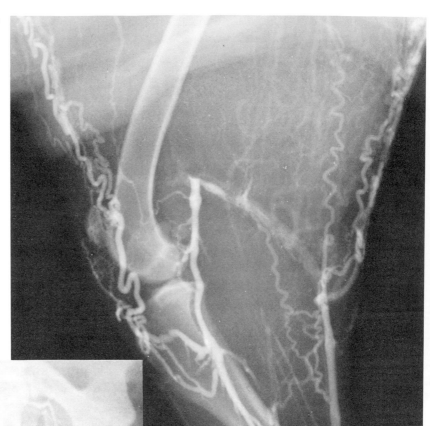

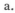

Fig. 6-1. (*above*) Venogram of the circulation in leg of dog with experimental fistula in the femoral vessels. Injection into vein of foot. Divergence of venous flow around the area of the fistula is shown. (*left*) Arteriogram. Prominent is the retrograde flow in vein distal to the fistula. (*opposite*) Diagram of arteriovenous circulation. Arteries cross hatched, veins stippled.

b.

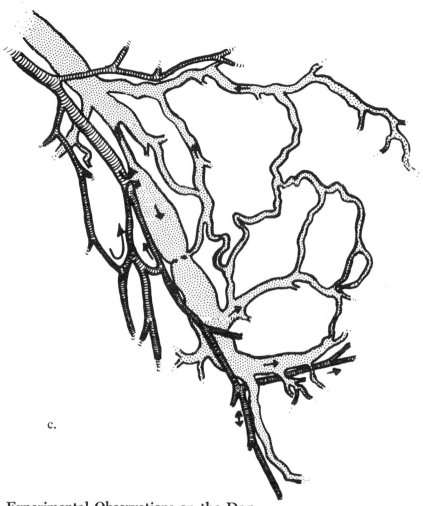

c.

Experimental Observations on the Dog

The circulation in a dog's leg with a experimental fistula is illustrated in the venogram shown in Figure 6-1. Just above the popliteal vein the centrally flowing blood is abruptly diverted by the stream of blood flowing retrogradely from the fistula and the dye is seen flowing away in a dilated collateral vein in lesser concentration because of the dilution. Still concentrated dye is seen flowing along the dilated superficial veins. Figure 6-1b shows the arteriogram, though the most striking feature of it is the marked

TABLE 6-1. EFFECTS OF EXPERIMENTAL A-V FISTULAE ON
BLOOD FLOW RATE *

	PROXIMAL ARTERY	DISTAL ARTERY	PROXIMAL VEIN	DISTAL VEIN
Acutely	1.1	– 0.2	1.0	– 0.2
After 4 months	1.7	– 0.8	0.9	– 1.4

* Blood flow rates in liters per minute. Retrograde flows are indicated by a (–) sign.

dilatation and incompetence of the valves of the femoral vein distal to the fistula. The artery proximal to the fistula is dilated; that distal to it, narrowed (in the arteriogram owing to the force of the injection the flow of blood in the distal artery appears to be in the normal direction). Figure 6-1c is a diagrammatic representation of the circulation in a limb with an A-V fistula. Arteries and veins are distinguished and the direction of flow along them shown by arrows. At the periphery of the circulation field feeding the fistula the direction of blood flow along the vessels may fluctuate, flowing into the fistula when vascular resistance in the tissues is high, and into the tissues when it is low. The predominance of veins in the illustrations exemplifies an important clinical finding: dilatation and incompetence of veins distal to the fistula is a major vascular disturbance of an A-V fistula.

An example of the enlargement of a fistula is given by our measurements of the rates of blood flow through it and the blood pressure around it at the time it was made and after it had been in existence for four months.

In the space of 4 months following the creation of the fistula the flow through it had doubled and much of this increase was due to blood flowing *towards* the fistula from the distal artery, and *away* from it in the distal vein. This increase in retrograde flow is the result of augmentation of circulation through the collateral vessels; an A-V fistula is regarded as the most potent stimulus to the development of collateral circulation known.

Along with the changes in flow the changes in pressure shown in Table 6-2 occurred.

The pressure in the artery feeding an acute fistula is lowered because of the runoff of blood into the fistula; it is even more

TABLE 6-2. EFFECTS OF EXPERIMENTAL A-V FISTULAE ON
BLOOD PRESSURE *

	PROXIMAL ARTERY	DISTAL ARTERY	PROXIMAL VEIN	DISTAL VEIN
Acutely	105/10	50/35	11	50/38
After 4 months	165/105	73/45	1	25/15

* Pressure in mm. Hg.

severely reduced in the arteries distal to the fistula. The venous pressure is moderately increased in the veins which drain blood directly from the fistula into the great veins and is markedly increased in the veins distal to the fistula. The combination of low arterial pressure and high venous pressure results in inadequate perfusion of the tissues distal to the fistula and danger of gangrene. In the established fistula these effects are diminished. Compensatory changes in the general circulation result in an increase in central arterial pressure, and development of collateral arteries round the fistula result in increased pressure distal to it. Dilatation of the veins, with developing incompetence of their valves results in a reduction of distal venous pressure. These changes result in improvement of the circulation to distal tissues even though the volume of flow of blood through the fistula may be increased.

Usual changes in flow and pressure in the four limbs of an established A-V fistula are:

PROXIMAL ARTERY	DISTAL ARTERY
Increased flow and dilatation	Reversed flow
Increased systolic pressure	Decreased systolic pressure
Decreased diastolic pressure	Decreased diastolic pressure

FISTULA
Rapid flow
Murmur
Thrill

PROXIMAL VEIN	DISTAL VEIN
Increased flow	Retrograde flow and greatly increased pressure
Increased pressure	Dilatation and incompetent valves

These experimental findings are to be applied to the description of the circulation in a human limb affected by an A-V fistula. In the acute fistula the ischemia in the limb may be severe enough to cause gangrene, and prompt repair of the vessels may be required. When the fistula has been in existence for some time, collateral pathways have developed and the distal tissues are perfused adequately. In the case of a femoral A-V fistula the region affected by the collateral circulation may extend to the knee and beyond. Measurements of blood flow, either by plethysmograph or skin temperature show an increased blood flow in the distal portions of the limb. The question arises whether the greatly increased flow is entirely directed into the fistula, leaving the tissues relatively ischemic, or whether development of collateral circulation is excessive resulting in over perfusion of the tissues. The marked degree of retrograde flow into the fistula, both venous and arterial, seen in experimental A-V fistulae, is in favor of the first possibility. Also in favor of this is the recording of *reduced* skin temperature of the toes of the affected limb. Breakdown of the skin into ulcers is also given as evidence of tissue ischemia, but whilst this may be a factor in the ulcers associated with congenital A-V fistulae, in the chronic acquired fistulae venous stasis appears to be a more likely cause of skin breakdown. In favor of the second possibility is the observation that intermittent claudication is not a feature of chronic A-V fistula, and even more in favor is the increased growth of the limb when a fistula affects the limb before the epiphyses have closed. The question of partition of blood flow between fistula and tissues remains for further study.

DIAGNOSIS

There are many causes of A-V fistulae (Table 6-3) but, whatever the cause, certain diagnostic features are commonly found in association with the lesion. The most important is the characteristic murmur. This is accentuated during systole but does not disappear during diastole. It has a machinelike quality. It cannot be too strongly emphasized that cases of A-V fistula will be

TABLE 6-3. CAUSES OF ARTERIOVENOUS FISTULAE

	CONGENITAL
Commonest Form	Persistence of portion of primitive capillary network, or embryonic anastomotic channels

	ACQUIRED	
Injury		
Penetrating	Commonly knife, bullet, splinter of bone, glass, or shell	
Blunt	Pressure of tissue against bone, closed scalp injury, heavy pressure on limb, childbirth	
Iatrogenic	Intentional:	For hemodialysis
		To increase bone length in child's limb (now discarded)
		To improve collateral circulation (questionable proceeding)
		Temporally to prevent thrombosis in venous graft (experimental)
	Unintentional:	Removal of lumbar disc
		Vein puncture (usually femoral)
		Renal biopsy
		Mass ligature of vessels at nephrectomy or splenectomy
Arterial Disease		
	Mycotic aneurysm	
	Medial arteriosclerosis and atherosclerosis (Figs. 6-2 and 3)	
	Fibromuscular dysplasia (renal vessels)	
	Ehlers-Danlos syndrome	
Neoplasm		
	Renal carcinoma	
	Retroperitoneal sarcoma (sometimes)	
	Metastasis (very occasional)	

missed unless the possibility of the condition is kept in mind and the characteristic murmur sought. The following cases in my personal experience demonstrate this point.

Case 1 (See Fig. 6-2). A 70-year-old lady complained of recent onset of swelling of the left arm. On examination the left arm was edematous with congested veins up the supraclavicular fossa. Physicians and surgeons concurred that the most probable cause was malignancy. This probability was furthered when the radiologist interpreted a venogram (comparable to Fig. 6-1a) as showing "obstruction" of the subclavian vein. A neurologist provided the correct diagnosis of subclavian A-V fistula by hearing the "typical continuous machinery murmur" radiating widely in the left clavicular area.

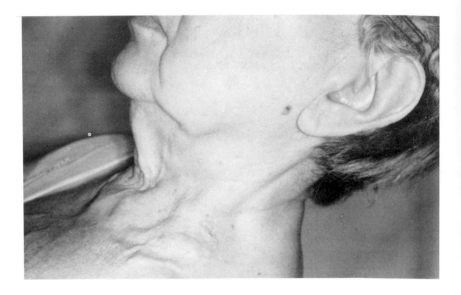

Fig. 6-2. Dilated supraclavicular veins in association with left subclavian arteriovenous fistula.

Case 2 (See Fig. 6-3). A 58-year-old man gave a history of three years of intermittent claudication in the left calf with coldness of the left foot. Arteriography showed an A-V fistula in the calf. A "typical continuous machinery murmur" was then heard over the calf. The patient could not recall any trauma which might have caused the fistula. He had obstructive arterial disease in both legs.

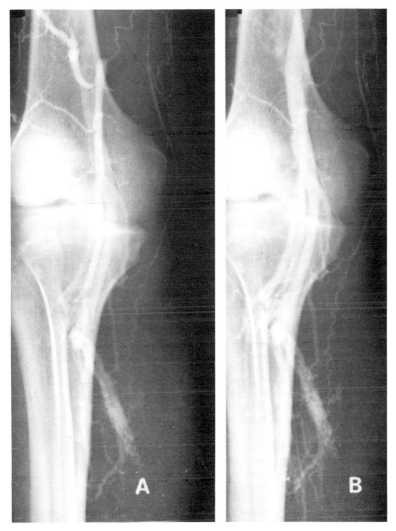

Fig. 6-3. Case 2. Arteriogram of femoropopliteal block and an arteriovenous fistula at the origins of the peroneal and anterior tibial arteries. (*A*) Early in the arteriogram the block at the femoropopliteal junction is shown, with filling of the popliteal artery by a well deveoped collateral. In the calf an abnormally dilated vein with retrograde flow is seen. The popliteal veins have filled early from the fistula, which is not clearly seen. (*B*) Venous stage of arteriogram.

Case 3. A 25-year-old man was admitted under the category of cardiac failure of unknown origin. His work-up included a measurement of cardiac output which was found to be inordinately increased. The consulting cardiologist applied his stethoscope, not only to the precordium, but to the sacrum posteriorally where the "typical continuous machinery murmur" was heard. Belatedly it was recognized that the venous congestion previously attributed to cardiac failure was particularly prominent in the left leg and left hypogastric region. The relevance of an operation for a prolapsed lumbar disc at the age of 21 in causing an occult A-V fistula was then recognized.

Case 4. A 65-year-old widow presented with the history of swelling of her left leg following the death of her husband 2 years previously. The appearance was of chronic deep venous thrombosis in that leg, but a "typical continuous machinery murmur" was heard in the left inguinal and iliac region. An arteriogram substantiated the diagnosis of left iliac A-V fistula.

Of all diagnostic procedures the single most important one is to use the stethoscope to listen for the characteristic murmur. A thrill may be felt over the artery if the vibrations within it are sufficiently forcible. Only in congenital A-V fistulae do exceptions to this rule occur, for the congenital fistula is often diffuse with multiple small channels over which no murmur is heard.

Dilatation of the artery supplying the fistula occurs and does not regress when the fistula has been excised. The sign is of little diagnostic value.

Venous dilatation and incompetence is a most valuable indication of A-V fistula. Unlike the incompetent veins associated with venous thrombosis the pressure in the veins into which an A-V fistula empties remains increased when the patient is recumbent. Failure of the veins to collapse when the limb is elevated may give rise to the suspicion of a fistula, and measurement of the venous pressure may be a useful diagnostic procedure.

Increased oxygen content of venous blood occurs with an A-V fistula, but since the oxygen content of venous blood varies over a wide range, this sign is of limited value.

Increased growth of the long bones may occur if the A-V fistula exists before the epiphyses close. The increased rate of growth apparently results from an increased supply of blood to the metaphysis in spite of the fistulous blood steal. Tibia and fibula are most often affected. Measurement of bone length is most accurately done from roentgenograms, though measurements from bony prominences usually suffice. A quick assessment of relative tibial length may be made in the office by having the patient sit with both feet squarely on the floor and observing the relative height of his knees. Fractures and Brodie's abscess are rare causes of discrepancy in the length of the long bones, and very rarely indeed one limb may be congenitally longer than its fellow.

Branham's sign is diagnostic of an A-V fistula. It is the prompt slowing of the pulse which occurs when a large fistula is temporarily occluded (Fig. 6-4). The sign may be elicited by com-

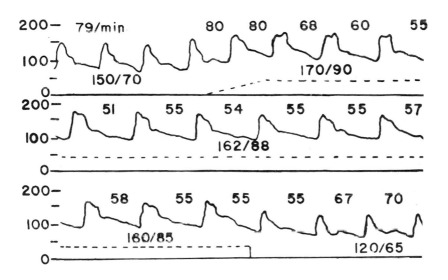

Fig. 6-4. Continuous recording of radial pulse during occlusion (dotted line) of a large femoral arteriovenous fistula. The pulse rate is calculated for each beat. The pulse slows promptly as systolic and diastolic pressures rise with the occlusion. On release of pressure the reverse changes are less prompt.

pressing the artery feeding the fistula or by occluding the circulation in the limb by means of a tourniquet. The sign is positive only when the flow through the fistula is large in comparison with a normal cardiac output. A fistula which produced this sign would be likely to be first recognized by murmur, thrill, and swelling, but the sign is not redundant for it is used to assess the size of the fistula and its effect on the circulation.

Increased skin temperature in certain circumstances may suggest the possibility of an A-V fistula. It is true that the limb with an A-V fistula is usually warmer than its fellow particularly in the region of the fistula, but the more distal regions may be cooler. A warmer limb particularly suggests an A-V fistula when the limb is swollen with the appearance of chronic venous incompetence.

Cardiac enlargement and increased cardiac output result from the circulatory demands of the fistula. The possibility that high output failure may be due to unrecognized A-V fistula should be recognized (See Case 3 above). Some of the enlargement of the heart is due to hypertrophy, but much is due to the increased stroke volume, and this portion regresses promptly when the fistula is closed.

CONGENITAL A-V FISTULAE

The anlage of the blood vessels go through such complicated transformations in their development that it seems remarkable that congenital A-V fistulae do not occur more often. Most fistulae in the extremities are small but slowly enlarge. A few are so extensive that they invade a whole limb. Their nomenclature is confusing.

They may be first recognized when a mother brings her baby for advice about a "birth mark," be it a port wine stain, a red stain or a pulsating hemangioma. Another method of presentation is when varicose veins develop in a limb with no obvious

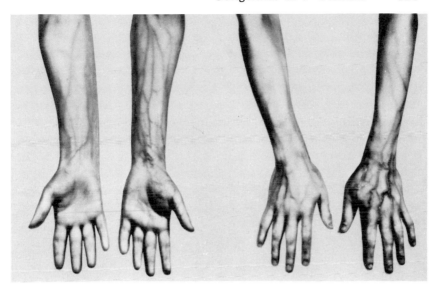

Fig. 6-5. Infrared photograph to show proliferation of subcutaneous veins of the left hand and forearm of a housewife
with a congenital arteriovenous fistula of the left thenar eminence. Surgery was not advised.

cause, particularly if the limb is warmer than its fellow (Fig.
6-5). The increased length of the limb may be the first sign
noticed. Ulceration of the skin occurs more frequently in congenital lesions than in acquired ones. Usually definite pulsation
can be felt over the fistula, and over some a bruit can be heard,
but these signs are less common than in acquired fistulae. The
volume of blood passing through the fistulae is seldom sufficient
to affect the general circulation. Arteriograms may be helpful
in diagnosis and for making a decision on whether surgical
treatment is feasible.

Congenital fistulae are usually too diffuse to be wholly excised
so that treatment is usually only palliative. Advice on the use
of make-up may be of cosmetic advantage, for the skin lesions
are often a source of distress. Pressure support of the legs is
useful in preventing ulceration of the skin. Though surgical
treatment of congenital fistulae often requires multiple operations

and carries with it a danger that amputation may be required, it should not be ruled out. Occasionally the arteriograms will show a circumscribed lesion which can be excised. We once had the fortunate experience of finding that the fistula in the foot of a young girl which was thought to be congenital was in fact acquired and due to a splinter of glass. Excision was relatively easy.

ACQUIRED A-V FISTULAE

Acute

Unless the possibility of an arteriovenous fistula is considered when dealing with a wound it is quite possible that it may be missed. The amount of external bleeding may be small, particularly if the external wound is small. The hemorrhage may be contained in the tissues and most of the blood may flow directly into the vein. Coincident nerve damage should not divert attention from the possibility of vascular injury. Arterial damage is to be suspected if there was arterial bleeding at the time of injury and particularly if the affected limb is cold and with small pulses. Fullness of the veins or edema of the limb may give indication of the increase in venous pressure. The characteristic bruit may not be apparent until some days after the establishment of a communication between the artery and vein.

Established

As the ecchymoses, hematoma, and edema of the acute injury resolve, the characteristic murmur over the fistula may begin to be heard. The patient himself may call attention to a pulsatile swelling with "purring" in it. Differentiation of a false aneurysm from an A-V aneurysm may be difficult, but the distinction is less important to make than previously, since both should be explored and repaired. There is little reason for leaving a suspected fistula untreated for few spontaneously close, and most develop more collateral circulation making the subsequent resection more difficult.

Aorta-Vena Cava Fistula

It is to be expected that a short circuiting fistula between the aorta and the vena cava would be a lethal lesion, but a small fistula is compatible with life, though not with health and well being because of the tendency of the fistula to increase in size.

Following intervertebral disc surgery, aorta-vena caval- or iliac fistula is a recognized complication. The true incidence is not known, but some 50 cases have been reported. The fistula is likely to be between the aorta and vena cava if the laminectomy is at the L/3-4 level, and at the L/4-5 level the iliac vessels are in danger. The effects of the fistula may become apparent immediately or may not become obvious until some years later when the fistula has increased in size. Reasons for suspecting that damage has been done to major blood vessels at the time of surgery are: (a) periods of hypotension and shock, (b) low diastolic pressure on recovery, (c) a bruit may be heard at this stage but is not essential for diagnosis, and (d) increased venous pressure in the lower extremities. With reasonable grounds for suspecting damage, prompt exploration should be carried out, as the patient's condition may deteriorate abruptly. After the postoperative period, the indications that a fistula had formed and is now enlarging may be suspected from the finding that the legs are becoming swollen. If this is unilateral, it may be mistaken for venous thrombosis, but pulsation should be felt for in the engorged veins of the femoral triangle and lower abdomen, and the characteristic bruit must be listened for. Other cases may present as a steady progression of high output cardiac failure over the postoperative years (See Case 3 above).

The rupture of an abdominal aneurysm into the inferior vena cava is unusual and sometimes is not recognized before the emergency operation for ruptured aneurysm. Some idea of its frequency is given by the figures of Beall et al. (1962). Some 1400 abdominal aneurysms had been repaired in Houston at this time; 130 had been leaking at the time of operation but only four had leaked into the vena cava. With leakage of the aneurysm into the vena cava rapid progress of cardiac, hepatic, and renal failure may be expected with massive edema of the lower extremities. The characteristic murmur may be recognizable but cannot be expected to be prominent with systolic hypotension. Only one of the four patients reported by Beall et al. showed a profound fall of diastolic pressure, and maintenance of this pressure at 60 to 70 mm. Hg has been our experience. Prompt surgical treatment is required.

Treatment

If the fistula is neglected steady increase in its size will result and the veins draining it become incompetent. The increased flow through the fistula puts an additional strain on the heart and cardiac failure may ensue. Rarely, subacute endarteritis may develop in the fistula. Treatment is preferably surgical. The fistula may be closed and continuity of the artery and vein restored, if possible. The great vascularity of the region around the fistula often makes its repair a very difficult proceeding. One approach to the fistula is transarterial with venous bleeding controlled by pressure alone so that the venous hole may be closed from the artery with minimal disturbance of the venous system. The artery is then repaired, or it may be preferable to insert a graft to replace a portion of it.

REFERENCES

Beall, A.C. Jr., Colley, D.A., Morris, G.C., Jr. and DeBakey, M.E.: Perforation of arteriosclerotic aneurysms into inferior vena cava. Arch. Surg., 86:809, 1963.

Holman, E.: Abnormal Arteriovenous Communications. p. 249. Springfield, Ill., Charles C Thomas, 1968.

Roberts, B. and Holling, H.E.: Arteriovenous Fistulae. *In* Hawthorne, H.R. ed.: Vascular Surgery. Springfield, Ill., Charles C Thomas, 1965.

7

Amputation

At no time in the progress of his disease is a patient more in need of skilled advice and treatment by physician, surgeon and physiotherapist than from the time that he becomes aware that a leg, or a portion of a leg, may have to be removed. Even surgical textbooks and, especially those on vascular surgery, tend to deal with the subject briefly, if at all, because of the opinion that amputation indicates failure of all that a surgeon hopes to achieve for his patient.

Fortunately arterial surgery has progressed in recent years so that a smaller proportion of patients with arterial disease require amputation. Less acclaimed has been the progress in medical and surgical management of the patient who has to undergo amputation, progress which results in him suffering less pain, anxiety and disability than previously, and in being able to anticipate a greater chance of retuning to an active life. But still more is required.

The methods of preparing a patient for the psychological trauma of amputation require continuing consideration. Techniques of amputation require assessment of their value in terms of the proportion of patients who are subsequently returned to active life and the length of time taken to reach that goal. Progress in the design of prostheses should concern physicians and surgeons as well as the department of physiotherapy and rehabilitation.

INDICATIONS FOR AMPUTATION

Traumatic damage to soft tissues, nerves and blood vessels may necessitate immediate amputation of a limb, but consideration should always be given to the possibility that painstaking repair might provide a chance of survival of the limb. In the case of the hand shown in Figure 7-1 the chance was taken that surgical repair might salvage the extremity. Though subsequent mobility of the hand was limited, the patient was well satisfied with the result and able to return to work.

Ischemia severe enough to cause gangrene may be an indication for amputation, but an arteriogram may show an unexpected opportunity for arterial reconstruction even in a seemingly irreparable limb. Such reconstruction, even if does not save the limb, may result in a much more limited amputation. No patient shoud be passed over for arterial reconstruction on the grounds that he is too old or has too much associated disease. A useful arterial reconstruction is less traumatic and dangerous than an amputation, less physically and emotionally stressful, and the subsequent rehabilitation requires less effort. Even if the hope of reconstruction fails, the arteriogram helps to decide at which level the limb should be amputated.

Intractable pain with ischemia is one of the most pressing reasons for amputation and often leads the patient himself to ask for amputation. Infected gangrene, which is often called wet gangrene, is frequently associated with insulin-requiring diabetes, and is an indication for an energetic attack on the infecting organism and more so on the metabolic disorder predisposing to it. Wet gangrene can exist only if there is a blood supply sufficient to maintain survival of the tissues if the infection could be surmounted. Other patients with "dry" ischemic gangrene run a persistent illness and fever for which no cause other than the ischemic limb can be found. If adequate blood supply cannot be restored to the limb in these cases the toxic absorption is an indication for amputation.

Other reasons for amputation which arise from time to time are: chronic infested and debilitating ulceration, massive arteriovenous fistula, and severe chronic lymphedema.

DECIDING THE LEVEL OF AMPUTATION

To decide at which level a limb should be amputated requires a judgment balanced between the wish to retain as much limb as

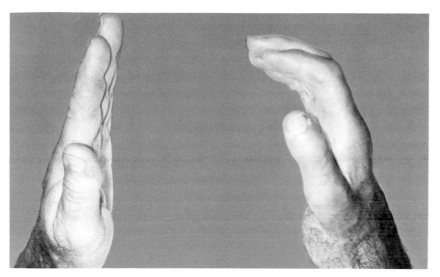

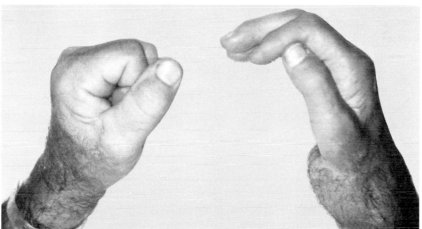

Fig. 7-1 (*Top*) Industrial machinery caused injuries to this man's right hand. The injuries included severance of radial and ulnar arteries, flexor tendons, median and ulnar nerves and crushing of the carpal bones. Continuity of the nerves and arteries was reestablished, with transplantation of tendons. Arterial thrombosis occurred but flow was reestablished by thrombectomy and heparinization. (*Bottom*) Eventually he achieved the degree of motion of his fingers shown in the above photographs. Three months after returning to work he developed carpal tunnel syndrome in the *left* hand, but this responded to the injection of steroids.

possible, the fear that the blood supply of the skin flaps will be inadequate for healing if the amputation is done too distally, and a knowledge of proper levels for the fitting of prostheses.

Most judgments of the viability of the skin flaps at the proposed level of amputation depend on clinical judgment of its "healthiness." The clinician bases this judgment on a number of impressions which are difficult to formulate. They include skin color and warmth, moistness, thickness and pliability, and the general condition of the patient is taken into account. Various objective aids to making this judgment have been suggested; skin temperature measurements, reactive hyperemia and histamine injection tests, venous filling time, blood flow measurements and the intensity of skin coloration when fluorescein is injected. None of these have come into general use, perhaps because they are superseded by the arteriogram.

The surgeon's judgment is also influenced by his experience with the operative technique which he plans to use. For example, when a below knee amputation has been decided on, an amputation with anterior-posterior flaps gives better cover for the ends of the bones. But if the blood supply is poor and the survival of the flaps seems in jeopardy, an amputation with lateral flaps may be preferable because they can be cut thicker and the geniculate collateral arteries are less likely to be damaged. The surgeon also has the opportunity to make a late judgment on the degree of bleeding which occurs as he cuts through the skin at the distal level.

The final decision of the level of amputation must rest with the surgeon, but the patient's physician may support the surgeon in making the decision and help to inform the patient of the reason for it. For these reasons the benefits and drawbacks of amputations at different levels are considered.

Above Knee

At the time when Sir Thomas Lewis wrote, it was the custom to amputate the leg through the lower third of the thigh "so as to make it reasonably certain that the amputation will be final." Amputation at this level may still be required for patients with acute obstruction at the aortoiliac level where for some reason arterial repair cannot be carried out, or it may be required when a femoropopliteal reconstruction has failed, or if there is reason to fear infection of the wound at a lower level. However, it is to be avoided if possible because:

1. A thigh stump, particularly a short one, makes it more difficult for the patient to turn in bed or sit up, so that he is more likely to develop hypostatic pneumonia or decubitus ulcer.

2. An older person finds it difficult to learn to use an above-knee prosthesis because of lack of flexion at the knee joint and the re-education of the sense of proprioception for a different manner of progression which is necessary.

3. The above difficulties are more liable to give rise to a state of depression and despair.

Below-Knee

Amputation below the knee is so preferable to amputation above the knee that in many cases in which an above-knee amputation seems inevitable, it is worth the surgeon's time to explore and attempt to reestablish flow in the distal superficial femoral and popliteal arteries before proceeding with the amputation. The exploration must be done through incisions so placed that they will not cut across the skin flaps of whatever amputation is decided on.

Compared to an above-knee amputation, the below knee offers the following advantages:

1. The immediate operative risk is less.

2. Following operation the patient is able to turn more easily in bed, to sit up without support, and even to get from bed to bathroom without assistance.

3. The patient's rehabilitation is less difficult in all regards.

4. If, as so often occurs, amputation of the other limb is subsequently required, the patient with a below knee amputation stands a better chance of retaining an active life.

Through-Knee

In recent years English surgeons have described the advantages of amputation through the knee joint. Operative mortality is reported to be lower, healing rapid, and since the patient becomes active sooner after operation, his reablement is quicker and more frequently successful. Prostheses suitable for this amputation are somewhat more expensive, but it would seem desirable to gain more experience with amputation at this level.

Syme's Amputation

When there is distal arterial occlusion, or when it has been possible to restore blood flow to below the knee but the fore-part of the foot is very ischemic, there may be sufficient circulation at the ankle to permit healing of an amputation just proximal to the ankle joint. If so a useful weight bearing limb results, but unfortunately the blood supply is often not adequate to permit survival of the extensively dissected heel flap of this amputation.

Transmetatarsal

Amputation through the fore-foot results in so little disability that this may be the preferred amputation when several foes are gangrenous. This amputation is indicated in severe digital ischemia whether due to emboli, thromboangiitis obliterans, or collagen vascular disease. It may occasionally be carried out when a perforating ulcer of the foot, due to neuropathy of diabetes mellitus, is resistant to healing.

Digital

Emboli, thromboangiitis obliterans, collagen vascular disease, diabetic gangrene, frostbite or trauma occasionally result in the need for amputation of a single toe. If a line of demarcation appears to be forming, it is often advisable to allow the toe to separate with a minimum of surgical intervention. Such treatment will result in greater preservation of tissue but slower healing.

PREPARING THE PATIENT

The fear that amputation may be required is a very common fear amongst patients with any disorder of their limbs, even if there are no grounds for such fear. If the physician is aware of the frequency of this fear he can get the patient to voice it and provide the necessary reassurance. When the condition of the limb is such that amputation becomes a possibility the patient must be carefully prepared for the possible event. Some patients who know amputees who live an active life have a more reasonable attitude themselves to the possibility. Others who know of patients who have died when undergoing amputation, or else are terrified of the disfigurement, may nourish an unreasoning fear of life, or death, with one limb missing.

It is seldom that doctor and patient can communicate on the subject until some definite event occurs such as a breach of the skin of the foot, or the need of an arteriogram. If the possibility of amputation is a real one it may be introduced by some phrase such as "this will show us whether we can save the foot or toe." Depending on the patient's reception of the idea the facts of amputation should be considered as fully as possible, but throughout it must be perfectly clear that every effort is being made to save the limb.

When surgeon and patient have agreed that an amputation is necessary, the operation should be carried out as speedily as possible because for most patients the period of waiting is one of extreme emotional stress. In two cases I have seen perforation of a peptic ulcer to occur whilst awaiting amputation. These sorry events bring out forcibly the need for the patient's doctor to continue his care during this period. During it not only are analgesics required but good use of tranquilizers also.

Some patients will refuse permission for amputation in spite of the need for it and the most careful preparation. Coercion should not be attempted because the occasional determined patient will live with a dead limb in an incredible fashion and manage to get from bed to toilet without the assistance which would have been required if an amputation had been performed. Moreover, amputation is associated with a mortality from pulmonary embolus, myocardial infarction, and other causes which is sufficient to deter one from pressing it onto a reluctant patient.

A definitive amputation may become too hazardous in some

patients who are severely ill because of septic absorption from an ischemic foot. Formerly a temporary guillotine amputation would have been carried out, but it is now more usual to freeze the limb distal to a tourniquet by means of dry ice. Putrefaction ceases at the low temperatures obtained, and valuable time is provided during which the patient's general condition may improve. This procedure will allay pain, toxicity, and anxiety in a remarkable fashion.

POSTAMPUTATION CARE

Vigorous efforts should be made to cajole, force, or otherwise get the patient to start activity by the second postoperative day. If this can be done the major setbacks of pulmonary emboli and pressure sores are likely to be avoided. Particular attention should be paid to straightening the knee and hip, for if a joint is allowed to remain flexed for even such a short period as a week subsequent rehabilitation can be considerably delayed. An active physiotherapist is most helpful at this stage. In recent years a decided advance has been to fit a rigid plaster of Paris dressing over the stump at the time of operation. This application holds the formation of edema in check, and healing appears to occur more rapidly. The use of a pneumatic cuff over the stump has been suggested and would seem to have the additional advantage that it can be more easily removed for inspection of the wound. Provision is made for both these appliances to be used with a weight-bearing prosthesis, but the original enthusiasm for such early walking is being tempered by the realization that it may delay healing. It is likely to be advantageous to wait several weeks until the setup appears to be healed before subjecting it to the jarring and pressure of walking on it.

During the early attempts at walking a lightweight walker is to be preferred to crutches. An elderly patient finds it hard to manage crutches and may catch a tip on an object and fall. A walker with four rubber feet is more stable and may be used on stairs, using the two front legs when going up and the two back legs when coming down. Hazards such as throw rugs on slippery floors should be banished. By the time the patient comes to a rehabilitation center he should have been well prepared and eager for the fitting of his permanent prosthesis.

In the postoperative period many patients are distressed by phantom limb pains. Explanation and reassurance are usually sufficient to allay this distress. This is fortunate, since medication often does not give relief. Dimethyl sulfoxide or sympathectomy have each been advised, but I have experience of neither.

REFERENCES

Experience with Through-Knee Amputation

Eastcott, H.H.G.: Arterial Surgery. chap. 6. Philadelphia, J.B. Lippincott, 1969.

Howard, R.R.S., Chamberlain, J., and MacPherson, A.I.S.: Through knee amputation in peripheral vascular disease. Lancet, *2*:240, 1969.

Martin, P., Stuart, R., Maelor, T.E.: Gritti-Stokes amputation in atherosclerosis: a review of 237 cases. Brit. Med. J., *3*:837, 1967.

Early Ambulation in Postoperative Care

Little, J.M.: A pneumatic weight-bearing temporary prosthesis for below-knee amputees. Lancet, *1*:271, 1971.

Mooney, V., Harvey, J.P., McBride, E., and Snelson, R..: Comparison of post-operative stump management: plaster vs. soft dressings. J. Bone Joint Surg., *53*:241, 1971.

Part III

DISORDERS OF SMALL VESSELS

8

Digital Ischemia

PHYSIOLOGY

The circulation to the fingers and toes differs from that of the general body skin in being peculiarly adapted to serve the purpose of regulation of body temperature. The arteriovenous anastomoses in the skin of the fingers, the arteries of the limbs with their venae comites, and the subcutaneous network of veins in the forearms form a remarkable thermostatic device of the body. Under cold conditions all cutaneous vessels of the hands and forearms constrict. The arterial supply to the fingers almost stops, that to the hands diminishes greatly, and the subcutaneous network of veins in the forearm is constricted. Heat loss from this area is greatly reduced by this diminution in blood flow, it is further reduced by the heat exchange system of the radial and ulnar arteries and their venae comites (Fig. 8-1). Having flowed through the cool tissues of the hands, chilled blood returns by the peri-arterial venae comites rather than by the surface veins. Heat passes from the arterial blood into the venous system thus simultaneously precooling arterial blood and rewarming venous blood. This counter current of heat transfer between artery and vein in cold conditions can generate temperature gradients of 0.35°C/cm. so that the arterial blood reaching the hand may be cooled to 21°C.

When the body is hot, the vessels of the extremities dilate and the arteriovenous anastomoses of the skin of the fingers open. Digital blood flow increases greatly, and venous blood now returns through the superficial veins of the forearm (Fig. 8-1b). Some heat is lost from the hot digits; more is lost from the dilated cutaneous veins. Blood flow through the venae comites is relatively small with little cooling of peripheral arterial blood.

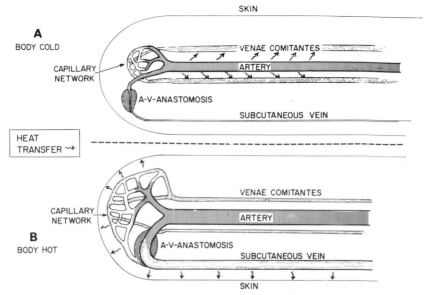

Fig. 8-1. Diagrams of circulation through fingers and forearm and direction of heat transfer under cold and hot conditions. When the body is cold, heat is conserved (*A*) and heat is lost when the body is hot (*B*).

The most remarkable organs in this system are multiple cutaneous A-V anastomoses of the digits. First described by Sucquet in 1862, they should not be confused with the arteriolovenous channels (thoroughfare channels) of Zweifach, for they have a more highly developed muscular coat and nerve supply. These anastomoses are capable of increasing digital blood flow one hundredfold when vasoconstrictor tone is released. The digital blood flow through these channels is affected by nervous, humoral, and physical (thermal) influences, and their sensitivity is so exquisite that the flow through them varies with the phases of respiration. The fingers have therefore a dual blood flow: the capillary network which functions as the blood-tissue exchange system, and the A-V anastomoses for general body temperature regulation.

Because the capillary response is usually overwhelmed by that of the A-V anastomoses, it is poorly understood. Only recently has the functioning of each of the channels of this dual circulation been investigated. In order to separate measurements of blood flow through the two channels, Coffman used plethysmography to measure total fingertip flow, and radioactive uptake for capillary (or exchange) flow. The difference between these measurements represents the flow through the A-V anastomoses. Measurements of flow rates in 10 normal subjects in warm and in cool environments provided figures which showed a decided reduction of A-V shunt flow on exposure to the cool environment and an insignificant reduction in capillary flow:

	TOTAL FLOW 100%	CAPILLARY % OF TOTAL	A-V SHUNT % OF TOTAL
In warm room (28°C)	59.7 ± 11.5 ml/100 ml/min	16	84
In cool room	32.7 ± 9.5 ml/100 ml/min	22	78

The important finding here is that flow required for nutrition of the tissues remains fairly steady, whilst flow subserving maintenance of body temperature fluctuates with environmental conditions. Of particular interest will be a comparison of neural and pharmacological agents on the two channels.

He investigated a group of patients with digital ischemia: 6 with sclerodactylia, 5 with rheumatoid disease, one with signs of thoracic outlet syndrome, and 12 with no discoverable cause for their symptoms. As a group they had a significantly lower capillary flow, in both warm (6.4 vs. 10 ml/100 ml/min) and cool (4.0 vs. 7.0) rooms, than did normal subjects. This finding quantitates the reduction in capillary flow indicated by the cyanosis or pallor of the digital skin in these patients and suggests that it is prolonged reduction in capillary flow to which nutritional changes in the fingers are due.

RAYNAUD'S PHENOMENON AND DISEASE

"Clinical medicine involves the continual effort to extract patterns from what was previously a continuum without blinding oneself to the clinical features which obstinately refuse to fit any of these patterns." *

The continuum of Raynaud's Disease arose in Raynaud's own account which described spasmodic discoloration of the digits and symmetrical gangrene of the fingers as a specific malady caused by overaction of the vasomotor center. In spite of the greater understanding of causes of digital ischemia which has developed since that time, the continuum of "Raynaud's Phenomenon" and "Raynaud's Disease" persists to perpetuate confusion and misunderstanding. A start to better understanding could be made by substituting "digital ischemia" as the collective term.

Raynaud's phenomenon is a spasmodic contraction of arteries and small arteries of the fingers leading to slowing or cessation of blood flow. It is provoked by exposure to cold and sometimes by emotion. The affected fingers are pallid or cyanosed when cold, and red and painful during the recovery phase (Fig. 8-2). Attacks of this phenomenon may be prolonged and the ischemia becomes severe enough to lead to nutritional changes in the ends of the fingers. At this stage the condition might be called Raynaud's disease.

"Raynaud's phenomenon" implies that digital arteries normal in structure overreact to constrictor stimuli. In "Raynaud's disease" structural abnormality of the vessels may be present. The distinction between the two cannot be clear-cut, for a digital artery may be narrowed by an organic lesion to a degree which does not interfere with flow when the vessel is normally dilated, but when the vessel is moderately constricted closure of the vessel results (Fig. 8-3). This vessel would appear to react to constrictor stimuli excessively. The toe shown in Figure 8-4 would be said

* Bannister, Roger: Lancet, 2:175, 1971

Fig. 8-2. (*Top*) Raynaud's phenomenon in a healthy man, age 31 years. Spasm in index, middle, and ring fingers on right hand after he had walked around the block on a cold day. He was lightly clad and his left hand was covered by a glove, his right hand was bare. (*Bottom*) Four minutes later the spasm remains in only the terminal portions of the middle and ring fingers of the right hand.

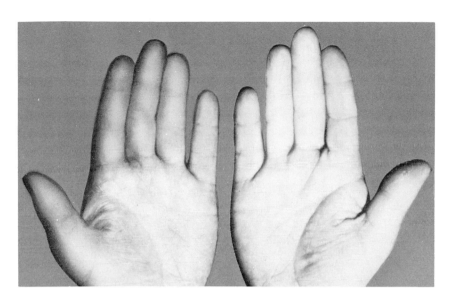

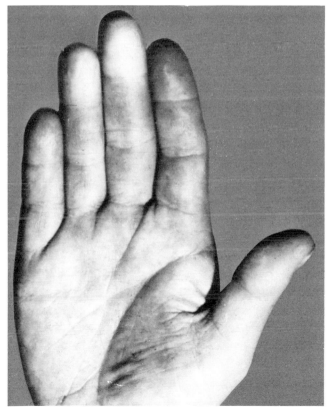

NORMAL ARTERY   PARTIALLY OBSTRUCTED
                                           ARTERY

DILATED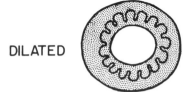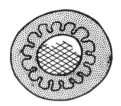

MODERATE
CONSTRICTION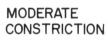

Fig. 8-3. Diagram of transverse section of normal and partially occluded arteries in the dilated and constricted states. The partially occluded artery is completely occluded with moderate constriction and might give the appearance of being "in spasm."

by many to exhibit Raynaud's phenomenon, for at the time of the photograph the toe was at heart level and was blue. If it had been elevated above heart level it would have been white. This is not the intermittent spasmodic arterial constriction of Raynaud's phenomenon; it is the cyanosis of persistent ischemia. Even if the patient were to be thoroughly warmed, her toe would remain cold and cyanosed, and if the toe were warmed directly she would be likely to experience pain rather than relief.

It must be recognized that patients exist whose "digital ischemia" obstinately refuses to fit into a definite pattern but whenever possible the existing pattern should be recognized. For example, it was important for the surgeon whose hands are shown in Figure 8-2 to know that he did not have to expect symmetrical gangrene to develop in his fingers. In a less fortunate case (Fig. 8-4) it was important to recognize that a general arterial disease existed to account for the ischemia. If "Raynaud's disease" is to

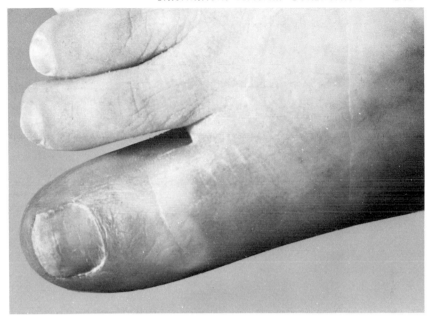

Fig. 8-4. Persistent ischemia with pallor and cyanosis in the toe of a female, age 43, with polyarteritis nodosa.

be used as a diagnosis, it should be recognized as an interim one to be used only until a more exact description of the vascular disease can be given. To use "Raynaud's disease" as a portmanteau term to cover a group of patients with digital ischemia of different etiologies perpetuates the century-old muddle originating in Raynaud's account. When persistent digital ischemia in a patient is found to be secondary to a systemic disease, it is always better to use the correct diagnostic term. If the best definition possible is desirable in clinical practice, it is essential in investigation of disease.

INTERMITTENT ARTERIAL CONSTRICTION

Raynaud's Phenomenon

Restriction of the blood flow to the fingers is a normal response to cold or emotion. Many people experience the nuisance of cold

CAUSES OF DIGITAL ISCHEMIA

INTERMITTENT DIGITAL ISCHEMIA (Raynaud's Phenomenon)
Provoked by cold and emotion

Exacerbated by
1. Activities causing repeated minor trauma to fingers: piano playing, typing, computer, pneumatic hammer or drill, hand scraping of reaction chambers.
2. Occupations associated with cold injury: telephone repair man or cold storage worker
3. Chronic disuse
Reflex sympathetic dystrophy, and central and peripheral nerve lesions.

PERSISTENT DIGITAL ISCHEMIA

Primary
4. Raynaud's disease
Digital artery thrombosis

Secondary
5. Arterial disease
Thromboangiitis obliterans
Arteriosclerosis obliterans (rarely)
6. Emboli
From heart, thoracic outlet, atheromatous aorta or subclavian artery
7. Arterial thrombosis
Trauma: mechanical, including occupations listed in (1) above; iatrogenic, as in arterial. catheterization.
Disorders of blood: polycythemia, primary and secondary thrombocythemia
Cryoagglutinins, globulins and fibrinogens
Possibly, homocystinuria
8. Systemic disease: progressive systemic sclerosis (acrosclerosis, scleroderma), disseminated lupus erythematosus, periarteritis nodosa, dermatomyositis
9. Intoxications: ergot, lead, arsenic, methysergide maleate
10. Doubtful connection. Primary pulmonary hypertension, Pheochromocytoma

---

numb fingers when driving an automobile on a cold morning. Possibly such spasm of the digital arteries—as Hunt described in himself many years ago—could be provoked in all subjects if the body were chilled and the fingers subjected to cold. Though Raynaud's phenomenon appears readily in susceptible persons, experimental production of it is difficult. Lewis gives a full account of the difficulties, particularly the vasodilator reaction which is likely to supersede the phenomenon when the hands are placed in iced water. The attacks shown in Figure 8-2 were provoked by walking lightly clad in cold weather.

The incidence of Raynaud's phenomenon in the general population is not known. Clearly its manifestations will be more frequent in cool temperate climates, as in the British Isles, where efforts to maintain a warm indoor temperature are thought to be unnecessary. It will be less frequent either in warmer climates or where the extreme cold compels people to take full protection. Contrary to what is usually stated, men, in comparable circumstances, appear to be as susceptible to it as women. The appearance of the phenomenon in a young man is not therefore more of an indication of associated disease than it is in a young woman. The surgeon whose hands are shown in Figure 8-2 was without complaints 3 years afterwards and suffered no inconvenience if he took suitable measures to keep warm.

When a patient complains of cold dead fingers, his concern may be quickly allayed if the doctor can assure him promptly that his condition is but an exaggeration of a normal response and that there is no need for him to be subjected to the emotional and monetary expense of a "collagen disease workup." To do this with confidence the physician requires that there be no sign of underlying arterial disease. There should be: (a) cessation of symptoms in warm weather and surroundings; (b) absence of nutritional changes in the skin of the digits; (c) presence of all peripheral pulses, including the digital when the subject is warm; and (d) evidence of normal circulation to the hands when tested by Allen's test.

After reassuring the patient the physician gives advice on keeping both body and fingers warm at all times. If, as so often happens, the female patient chooses to follow the fashion designer rather than the physician in her choice of dress, the disappointed physician can find sympathy in Lewis' comment on acrocyanosis: "It came in with short skirts and will go out with them."

Attempts to treat Raynaud's phenomenon by drugs or surgery are unlikely to be successful, and they are liable to convince the patient that she has a disease that needs treatment, rather than an exaggeration of a normal response to cold which can be avoided simply by keeping warm. Raynaud recognized that precaution rather than treatment was required: "syncope and local asphyxia in the simple state . . . dead fingers . . . constitute scarcely a slight inconvenience, which often passes unperceived so that it does not require any treatment."

Raynaud's Phenomenon and Vibrating Tools. Raynaud's phenomenon as an industrial disease was first reported in 1911 and has since been associated with the use of high-speed vibrating tools in cool conditions. A recent Hungarian study estimated that after ten years' use of pneumatic hammers only 10 per cent of steel cast fettlers remained free from complaints of Raynaud's phenomenon. The disorder has been less frequent in the United States, since work places have been kept warmer in winter. The British Industrial Injuries Advisory Council recently advised that "vibration induced white fingers" should not be regarded as an industrial injury, for which compensation could be awarded, on the grounds that it would be extremely difficult to establish a clear connection between a significant and sufficient duration of industrial exposure and the appearance of Raynaud's phenomenon. It was generally agreed that the disorder is a minor one.

Repeated trauma to the hands in certain manual occupations may lead to localized thrombosis in portions of the arterial system of the hand. This may be an occasional cause of digital artery thrombosis (see below) and chronic digital ischemia.

Acrocyanosis, Chilblains, and Pernio. Acrocyanosis is related to Raynaud's phenomenon in that it is manifested by attacks of coldness and blueness in the hands when exposed to cold. The condition occurs mainly in young women with habitually cold and sweaty hands. When the hands are cold they are cyanosed; on warming they flush to a bright red and give rise to a sense of heat. The skin usually shows little change, but chilblains may develop on the knuckles. Lewis' studies indicated that whereas in Raynaud's phenomenon the constriction was in the digital arteries, in acrocyanosis it was in the small arteries or arterioles of the hands. This condition was always a rarity in this country, but common in the British Isles where the indoor temperature is usually kept about 10°F lower than in the U.S.A.

A chilblain is a form of chronic inflammation due to cold. It consists of a subcutaneous nodule of small round cells over which the cyanosed skin is thinned and may break down giving rise to an indolent and painful ulcer.

Pernio describes both conditions and was used to describe the condition in limbs paralyzed by anterior poliomyelitis.

Vasospasm of Disuse. The warmth of a limb is naturally maintained by the exothermic reactions of active muscles. With inactivity circulation through the muscles diminishes, and in cool surroundings the limb becomes cold. The small arterial inflow is cooled by the venae comites and by passing through cool muscles, so that blood reaching the hands and feet is already chilled. Raynaud's phenomenon may result, but the more usual appearance associated with chronic inactivity is that of pernio or acrocyanosis. The more common causes of chronic disuse are anterior poliomyelitis, traumatic denervation, cerebrovascular accidents, and reflex sympathetic dystrophy.

At an early stage the arterioles of a limb with vasospasm from disuse will dilate fully when the subject becomes warm, but with long continued disuse and exposure to cold, atrophic changes proportional to the extent and duration of the disuse gradually occur. The natural wrinkles over the knuckles tend to smooth, the fingers taper, the pulp atrophies, and the nails curve and thicken. Breaks in the skin due to minor trauma become painful and heal with difficulty. Over the limb as a whole the venules of the skin lose tone and dilate, even becoming telangiectatic. Lymphatic drainage slows and the legs particularly develop edema readily. These changes occur with disuse, even with preservation of motor and sensory innervation; it is not necessary to introduce ideas of "vasomotor disturbance" or lack of "trophic factors". Though sympathectomy may effect an improvement in circulation in some cases of disuse of the legs, to keep the limb warm at all times would be simpler and more effective.

Cold Agglutination Syndrome. Circulating cold agglutinins are a rare cause of digital ischemia. Cold agglutinins are macroglobulins capable of causing aggregation of red cells at temperatures below 37°C. They are most active at 0° to 5°C, but sera with high titers commonly show activity at 20° to 25°C, which is a range of temperature to which fingers in a cold or temperate climate are commonly subjected. In patients with such high titers cooling of the fingers to these temperatures has been shown to result in a cessation of blood flow through them. Warming the fingers customarily reverses the agglutination promptly and restores blood flow with no apparent residual vascular injury, but prolonged cooling may result in irreversible changes in the fingers, ears, nose tip, or other exposed parts.

Low levels of cold agglutinin activity are commonly present in healthy persons, but patients with digital ischemia from this cause may be expected to have titers in excess of 1:1,000 and even titers of 1:100,000 have been observed. Such patients have chronic hemolytic anemia and episodes of hemoglobinuria. If the condition is secondary to carcinoma lymphoma, or other malignant disease, as it usually is, the digital ischemia is usually a very secondary phenomenon.

Cryoglobulins have also been implicated in production of Raynaud's phenomenon, as have cryofibrinogens. In the majority of patients with digital ischemia from these causes the disease responsible for the abnormality of plasma proteins is obvious, whether it be multiple myeloma, primary macroglobulinemia, or other lymphoid malignancy. Very rarely no cause may be found to the cryoglobulinemia when the patient falls into the category of "essential cryoglobulinemia."

Treatment is by avoidance of cold, for though penicillamine inactivates the agglutination properties of the macroglobulin responsible for cold agglutination, its use is not practical for long term management of the disorder.

PERSISTENT DIGITAL ISCHEMIA

Reasons for the suspicion that organic and permanent changes have taken place in the digital circulation of a patient with complaint of coldness of the fingers are:

1. Coldness of the hands and numbness of the fingers which occurs in warm and comfortable surroundings, and in the warmer months of the year.

2. First appearance of symptoms in middle age.

3. Unilateral symptoms.

4. Atrophy of the pulp of the distal phalanx with tapering of the finger and hardening and thinning of the skin of the distal phalanx. Appearance of cracks and ulceration of the skin alongside the fingernail.

5. Slowness of return of color to one or more fingers when Allen's test is performed.

6. Absence of one or more digital pulses when the hand is warm or of radial, ulnar, or thenar space pulsation.

7. Diminished response to the vasodilatation test.

Raynaud's Disease

If any form of digital ischemia should be termed "Raynaud's disease," it is the chronic occurrence of Raynaud's phenomenon. The patient is usually a middle-aged woman who has had cold fingers for many years and Raynaud's phenomenon since puberty. The skin on the ends of her fingers is dry and hard and when compressed with the examiner's fingers gives a sensation described as eggshell crackling. There may be small scars on the fingertips, cracks, and even ulceration alongside the fingernail (Fig. 8-5). Symptoms disappear when the warmer weather occurs, only to return the next winter. Women with this condition go on for years without becoming noticeably worse, or better, and if they are typists, computer workers or musicians, they suffer restricted digital dexterity. It is remarkably difficult to get these

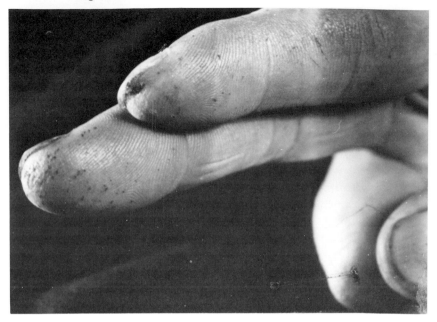

Fig. 8-5. "Raynaud's Disease." Hardening and pitting of skin of distal phalanges with small ulcer on the forefinger and atrophy of the finger pad.

patients to take simple measures to keep themselves warm. One might suspect that the disorder is less hyperreactivity to cold and more lack of appreciation of reduction in temperature, so that vascular reaction to cold precedes the awareness of it.

Digital Artery Thrombosis

Raynaud described symmetrical gangrene of the fingers and Lewis described bilateral gangrene of the digits in the young and in the elderly. Some of these cases may have been examples of obstruction of one or more of the digital arteries as shown in Figure 8-6. The patient is often a man in late middle age, (though women are also affected), who has been free of Ray-

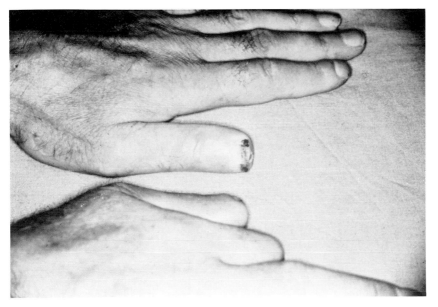

Fig. 8-6. Digital artery thrombosis; loss of distal phalanges of thumbs and right index finger. Male patient, age 56, six months after start of symptoms.

naud's phenomenon or digital ischemia when, without any obvious cause, over a period of a few days the thumb or index finger of one or both hands becomes severely ischemic or gangrenous. Remarkably, the circulation to the digits as shown by skin temperature or plethysmographic studies is normal to the border of the gangrene. Arteriography shows obliteration of the involved arteries (Fig. 8-7). Subsequently other fingers may be similarly involved. The clinical picture suggests local arterial thrombosis; no cause has yet been discovered. Except for the localized gangrene the prognosis is usually good.

The abrupt onset, equal incidence in men and women, and the localization of the ischemia distinguish this condition from Raynaud's disease. Some descriptions, notably Lewis', do not distinguish this form of digital ischemia from the gangrene of the fingers, toes, ears, and nose which may occur in a terminal illness. The condition of the patients makes this distinction clear.

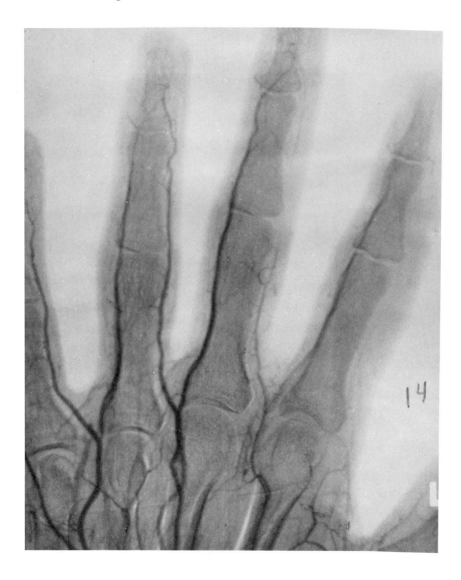

Fig. 8-7. Arteriogram of patient with digital thrombosis showing: abrupt block of digital artery on the thenar aspect of index and middle fingers, normal arterial supply to ring and little fingers.

Another diagnosis to consider is embolism. Embolism in the arm is not common but may occur from a thoracic outlet cause, or the dislocation of a plaque of atheroma, or from a mural thrombus following a myocardial infarct, or from left atrial thrombus in mitral stenosis and atrial fibrillation. In embolism a sudden widespread ischemia narrows as collateral circulation takes over, whereas in digital artery thrombosis the ischemia increases over a matter of days.

Undoubtedly many of these patients are diagnosed as having thromboangiitis obliterans. They differ in that the arterial thrombosis is sharply localized in the digital artery whereas in thromboangiitis obliterans by the time gangrene occurs the radial and ulnar and radial arteries are likely to have been involved. Digital artery thrombosis also differs from thromboangiitis obliterans in that it affects women, it is not closely associated with cigarette smoking, and affects neither the veins nor the arteries of the legs.

Ergotism

Though ergotism is rare, it is of considerable interest, first because of its historical background, secondarily because of the unusual mechanism which results in gangrene, and thirdly because recognizing an obscure vascular disease as being due to ergot provides a most satisfying event in a physician's professional life.

The patient is often unaware that he is taking a medical preparation containing ergot, but thinks of it as being for headache, or to procure an abortion. The medication is often taken by suppository which may lead the patient to deny that he is taking any "pills." The vascular symptoms have been preceded by paresthesias, sensory impairment and burning pains. These are followed by cramps with attacks of coldness, numbness with pallor and marbling of the skin. If arteriography is done at this stage, remarkable segmental lengths of spasm may be seen, or a length of an artery such as the radial may be in threadlike spasm. If these early symptoms are not recognized, the skin begins to break down by bruises or blisters, and over a period of weeks the dry gangrene of ergotism follows. The lower limbs are more often affected than the hands, and the gangrene is associated with burning pain until the tissue drys and shrivels.

Cervical Rib and Thoracic Outlet Syndromes

A *cervical rib* or abnormally high first rib may be the cause of vascular or neural disorders in the arms. Vascular symptoms result from compression of the subclavian artery between the upper and anterior surface of the rib and the clavicle, neural symptoms from stretching the lower cords of the brachial plexus over a high incomplete cervical rib. Seldom therefore, do vascular and neural manifestations coincide, though numbness and tingling, and even muscular wasting are features of both and may suggest a coincidence.

The diagnosis of one case of cervical rib was made in an unusual manner. A first year medical student was referred as a case of "Raynaud's disease." Since starting her medical course she had continued to take pleasure in playing the organ. She had noticed, however, that while playing the organ in a cool church her left arm began to ache and the fingers of that hand became numb and cold. She found that abducting her left arm resulted in disappearance of her radial pulse and concluded that her left subclavian artery was being compressed by a cervical rib. Her diagnosis proved to be correct and the removal of the rib resulted in disappearance of her symptoms.

This history illustrates some features of digital ischemia due to a cervical rib. The patient is usually a woman in the late twenties or thirties; the ischemia is usually unilateral and affected by the position of the arm with respect to the shoulder girdle. Most cases are not diagnosed until the trauma of continued compression results in formation of thrombus in the artery from which emboli arise. Permanent ischemia, or even gangrene of the fingers may result from neglect of early symptoms. On palpation the anterior end of the rib can sometimes be felt above and behind the clavicle, the pulsation of the subclavian artery is felt above this, especially if postcompression aneurysmal formation has occurred. The radial pulse may disappear with the arm in different

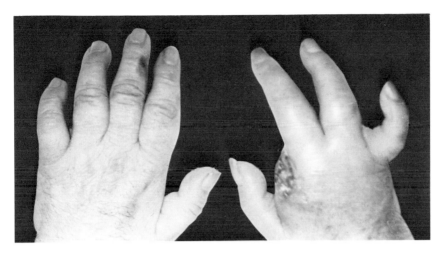

Fig. 8-8. Ischemia and loss of fingers of right hand. Pressure from the use of a crutch had thrombosed the right axillary artery, and emboli had further blocked the brachial vessels.

positions and simultaneously a bruit may be heard over the point of compression. X-ray demonstrates the cervical or high first rib.

Crutch Pressure. Figure 8-8 illustrates the result of the use of a crutch for many years. The mechanism of the vascular changes in the hand are the same as those of cervical rib, except that the section of artery which is compressed is the axillary. This complication does not occur until the crutch has been used for many years. The patient was an overweight and unintelligent victim of poliomyelitis. He had no palpable arterial pulsations in his right arm because of thrombosis extending from the axillary artery. Treatment included removal of the gangrenous tissues and attempts to train him to use a walker which did not compress the axillary artery.

Thoracic Outlet Syndromes. Cervical rib and crutch pressure are two well defined causes of arterial compression at the thoracic outlet. Other causes are less distinct. In the absence of a cervical rib or use of a crutch, vascular disorders may result from compression of the subclavian artery between clavicle and high first rib; between scalenus anticus and medius muscles or on a fibrous aponeurosis of the former muscle; or over a fibrous band representing a rudimentary cervical rib.

It is usually difficult to decide at which point compression is occurring, and even at operation doubt may still exist because recumbency and muscular relaxation alter the relationships. Arteriography with the arm in different positions which give rise to symptoms may determine the point of compression.

Carpal Tunnel Syndrome. Compression of the median nerve in the carpal tunnel results in pain, paresthesia and numbness of the first three digits with wasting of the muscles to the thumb. The symptoms may occasionally suggest digital ischemia from a thoracic outlet syndrome, and occasionally Raynaud's phenomenon occurs in the affected fingers. This account is therefore given here though the syndrome is essentially the result of compression of a peripheral nerve, and the explanation given for the occurrence of Raynaud's phenomenon is that denervation of the digital vessels has rendered them more susceptible to cold.

Typically the patient complains of unilateral, sometimes bilateral paresthesia of part or all of the distribution of the median nerve in the hand (the thumb, index and middle fingers); the discomfort may awaken the patient from sleep. In obscure cases the discomfort may strike up the arm as well as in the hand, giving rise to a suspicion of neurovascular compression at the thoracic outlet. There may be some wasting of muscles of the thenar eminence and diminished sensation of the area of median supply in the hand. Tinel's sign, a sensation of tingling in the median distribution when the wrist is extended and percussion made over the transverse carpal ligament is useful. Nerve conduction measurements showing delayed conduction velocity over the median nerve at the wrist are diagnostic.

When the diagnosis is made, the possibility of an underlying condition causing swelling of connective tissue should be considered: myxedema, amyloidosis, pregnancy, myeloma have been implicated.

Treatment is by splinting of the wrist at night and by injection of hydrocortisone into the carpal tunnel. In resistant cases, surgical resection of the flexor retinaculum and removal of excess connective tissue will afford relief.

GENERAL ARTERIAL DISEASES ASSOCIATED WITH DIGITAL ISCHEMIA

General arterial diseases which may give rise to digital ischemia are: thomboangiitis obliterans, systemic lupus erythematosus polyarteritis nodosa, systemic progressive sclerosis, dermatomyositis, rheumatoid arthritis, and blood dyscrasias. Digital ischemia is usually an incident in the course of these diseases, with the exception of systemic sclerosis (sclerodactylia) the symptoms of which may be localized to the fingers for many years. Those diseases are described in the next chapter.

When one of these diseases is suspected to be present the physician should turn his attention to the possible manifestations of systemic disease: intermittent fever, arthralgia, myalgia, cutaneous rash, urticaria, peripheral neuropathy, dyspnea. Investigations may show anemia or polycythemia or thrombocythemia, elevated sedimentation rate, false positive serological reactions, dysproteinemia, proteinuria, or microscopic hematuria.

TREATMENT OF DIGITAL ISCHEMIA

General

To avoid the vasoconstrictor stimulus of cold the patient should maintain the indoor temperature of her house at 75°F. In the morning a hot bath is a good way to start the day with a store of body heat. Time should also be allowed to run the engine of the automobile for long enough for the heater to start functioning. Clothing should be warm to the point of discomfort and thick woolen or fur gloves and lined boots are to be worn out of doors. Gloves heated by electric battery or chemical means are available. Bed socks and gloves may be advisable at night. Cigarette smoking is forbidden as being strongly vasoconstricting. Those who are willing are well advised to spend the winter in a warmer climate. These simple and effective measures are usually disregarded, for the patient cannot realize their importance, even when it is pointed out to her that her symptoms abate during the warmer months, and that a trial of such simple means is innocuous and inexpensive.

Vasodilators

Alcohol is a cutaneous vasodilator and need not be forbidden. Tolazoline hydrochloride (Priscoline*) 80 mg. long acting tablets can be taken in the morning and may be helpful. Side effects are gastrointestinal irritation, arterial hypo- or hypertension, tachycardia and muscular tremor. Phenoxybenzamine (Dibenzyline†) 10 mg. is an adrenolytic agent and is given twice or three times a day. The side reactions of this drug are tachycardia, orthostatic hypotension, nasal congestion and headache. It must be admitted that the effect of vasodilator drugs is usually disappointing. Griseofulvin, 500 mg. tablet taken at night, has been said to diminish the reactivity of the digital arteries to cold and therefore act as a vasodilator.

During the last decade good effects have been claimed following intra-arterial injection of phenoxybenzamine, bretyllium, and reserpine. The last has been most often described recently: 0.5 mg. in saline is slowly injected into the brachial or radial artery. Often the injection is followed by up to 1.0 mg. of reserpine by mouth each day. It is reported that this treatment reduced the number and severity of the attacks of pain for as long as seven months, and if attacks occurred they could more easily be terminated. Side effects of the reserpine therapy: depression, hypotension, tachycardia and nasal stuffiness were found to be rare. No controlled trials of this therapy have been carried out, and indeed to do so might be difficult because of the systemic effects of the drug and because of the variety of diseases which have been lumped together under the eponym "Raynaud's disease."

* Trademark, Ciba Pharmaceuticals.
† Trademark, Smith, Kline & French.

Surgical

Cervical Rib and Thoracic Outlet Syndrome. When symptoms and signs indicate compression of the subclavian artery by a cervical rib the preferred treatment is removal of the abnormal rib. Use of the axillary approach, originally advocated by Goetz for sympathectomy and more recently by Roos for removal of the rib provides cosmetic advantages with less postsurgical discomfort. Surgery should be advised early rather than late to avoid the complications of arterial thrombosis and embolism and later aneurysmal formation. If the artery appears to have suffered permanent damage there is a good case for insertion of an autogenous vein graft to prevent further thrombosis and embolism. When thoracic outlet obstruction arises from causes other than a cervical rib, the probability of relief by surgical means is somewhat less certain. The patients are advised to perform exercises to strengthen the shoulder muscles, and if no improvement is apparent after months, surgical exploration of the region should be carried out.

Sympathetic Block and Denervation. To block the stellate ganglion by infiltration of local anesthetic is a simple procedure in practiced hands. We have found it useful in cases of painful necrosis of the fingertips. If the block results in warming of the hand and relief from pain, it may be repeated daily or on alternate days. In some cases the temporary relief will tide the patient over until collateral pathways are functioning freely. The procedure is also useful in reflex sympathetic dystrophy. If sufficient relief is obtained from the stellate block, cervicodorsal sympathectomy may be considered. Following this in successful cases there is an immediate warming of the hands. Unfortunately the results of cervical sympathectomy are not as permanent as those of lumbar sympathectomy, and a gradual cooling of the hands occurs over the next 9 months. The recurrence of symptoms after cervical sympathectomy has been attributed to incompleteness of the sympathectomy, a sensitization of the denervated vessels to vasoconstrictor substances, or a regrowth of sympathetic fibers. Whatever its cause, it has resulted in sympathectomy being seldom advised for chronic digital ischemia, as in Raynaud's disease or sclerodactylia.

REFERENCES

Circulation in the Fingers and Forearms with Reference to Heat Conservation and Loss

Bazett, H.C., et al.: Temperature changes in blood flowing in arteries and veins in man. J. Appl. Physiol., *1*:3, 1948.

Grant, R.T. and Bland, E.: Observations on arteriovenous anastomoses in human skin and in bird's foot, with special reference to the reaction to cold. Heart, *15*:385, 1931.

Sucquet, J.P.: D'une Circulation derivative dans les Membres et dans la Tete chez l'Homme. Paris, 1862.

Wilkins, R.W., Doupe, J., and Newman, H.W.: The rate of blood flow in normal fingers. Clin. Sc., *3*:403, 1938.

Raynaud's Phenomenon

Coffman, J.D. and Cohen, A.S.: Total and capillary finger-tip blood flow in Raynaud's phenomenon. New Eng. J. Med., *285*:259, 1971.

Hunt, J.H.: The Raynaud phenomena: a critical review. Quart. J. Med., *5*:399, 1936.

Lewis, T.: Experiments relating to the peripheral mechanism involved in the spasmodic arrest of the circulation in the fingers, a variety of Raynaud's disease. Heart, *15*:7, 1929.

Major, R.H.: Classic Descriptions of Disease. p. 480. Springfield, Ill., Charles C. Thomas, 1948.

Cold Agglutination Syndrome

Marshall, R.J., Shepherd, J.T. and Thompson, I.D.: Vascular responses in patients with high serum titers of cold agglutinins. Clin. Sci., *12*:255, 1953.

Thoracic Outlet Syndromes

Eden, K.C.: The vascular complications of cervical ribs and first thoracic rib abnormalities. Brit. J. Surg., *27*:111, 1940.

Falconer, M.A. and Waddell, G.: Compression of subclavian artery. Lancet, 2:539, 1943.

Holling, H.E.: The etiology of vascular symptoms occurring in cases of cervical rib. Guy Hosp. Rep., 89:285, 1939.

Rosati, L.M. and Lord, J.W.: Neurovascular compression syndromes of the shoulder girdle. *In:* Modern Surgical Monographs. New York, Grune and Stratton, 1961.

Treatment

Abboud, F.M., Eckstein, J.W., Laurence, M.S.: Preliminary observations on the use of intra-arterial reserpine in Raynaud's phenomenon. Circulation, 35:11, 1967.

Charles, R. and Carmick, E.S.: Skin temperature changes in Raynaud's disease after griseofulvin. Arch. Derm., 101:331, 1970.

Roos, D.B.: Experience with first rib resection for thoracic outlet syndrome. Ann. Surg., 173:429, 1971.

9

Various Vascular Diseases

A chapter on various vascular diseases presents a challenge to arrange them in a pattern which will be most useful in clinical practice. The clinician does not find it easy to do this because he thinks of his patients as individuals reacting in different ways to the diseases from which they suffer. The task becomes less difficult if the development of knowledge and technique permits one to emphasize one facet of the body's response to the disease. Thus in the nineteenth century arrangement of diseases according to their pathological and histological appearances resulted in a greater understanding of disease processes. At the present time increasing knowledge of the body's immunological responses appears likely to provide a comparable increase in understanding.

The classification of vascular diseases based on their pathological and histological appearances contributed greatly to our knowledge of them, but the fact that the nature of histological changes following a noxious stimulus to arterial tissues is limited and that all destructive processes will result either in obliteration of cellular pattern or its conversion to scar tissue limits the value of observations on pathological material. Failure to appreciate this limitation underlay the mistaken opinion that thromboangiitis obliterans did not exist as a distinct disease but was a premature manifestation of atherosclerosis. Histological investigation also led to the classification of a group of vascular diseases which had in common the pathological process of fragmentation, swelling, and destruction of the collagen fibers of the tissues surrounding the vessels. However, the concept of collagen vascular disease has not proved of lasting value in clinical practice and the category is falling into disuse.

It seems premature to base a classification on immunological reactions, although in recent years the immunological reactions associated with systemic lupus erythematosus have become more clearly defined, and those in rheumatoid arthritis illuminated, we have still much to learn of these mechanisms in other vascular diseases.

The following classification of vascular diseases by both histological and immunological processes, based on Zeek's * classification, provides a semblance of order into this disorderly subject. It is likely that any such classification will have to be modified as further study produces greater knowledge of these diseases.

NECROTIZING ANGIITIDES *

1. Periarteritis nodosa
2. Systemic "allergic" angiitis
3. Allergic granulomatosis
     (a) Loeffler's syndrome
     (b) Wegener's granulomatosis
4. Collagen vascular disease
     (a) Progressive systemic sclerosis (scleroderma)
     (b) Dermatomyositis
     (c) Systemic lupus erythematosus
     (d) Rheumatoid arthritis
     (e) Acute rheumatic fever
5. Giant celled arteritis
     (a) Cranial arteritis and polymyalgia rheumatica
     (b) Aortic arch arteritis (pulseless disease)
6. Arteritis following surgical correction of coarctation of the aorta

* Zeek, P.M.: Periarteritis nodosa. A critical review. Am. Jour. Clin. Path., *22*:77, 1952.

In the arrangement in this chapter I have tried to evade insistent requirements of histological or immunological classification of various vascular diseases in the hope that a rearrangement will stimulate fresh approaches to a difficult subject. I have adopted a classification which comes easily to a clinician, that is the seemingly simple one of primary vascular diseases and vascular diseases which are secondary to other diseases. This has been done with full recognition that we cannot be certain into which of these two categories certain diseases fall; we cannot state dogmatically that vascular phenomena are primary in progressive systemic sclerosis, nor that they are secondary in systemic lupus erythematosus. The value of any classification depends ultimately on the value of its application to clinical medicine, and a satisfactory classification of various vascular diseases is still required.

PRIMARY VASCULAR DISEASES

SCLERODERMA

Scleroderma (Sclerodactylia) is a systemic disorder with characteristic connective tissue and vascular alterations associated with the cutaneous manifestation of a hard, tight skin. The question of whether the disorder is primarily one of blood vessels or of connective tissue surrounding them remains unresolved.

The brunt of the disease may fall on the viscera with minimal digital ischemia; this form is called either systemic scleroderma or progressive sclerosis. It is a malignant disorder in which death occurs from renal or cardiopulmonary failure. Conversely digital ischemia may be a major manifestation when the disease may be termed acrosclerosis or sclerodactylia. In this form of the disease visceral involvement is relatively light, and the course is chronic. Intermediate forms occur but it is usual for a case to fall into one category of progressive systemic sclerosis, and the remainder are examples of sclerodactylia. The following description emphasizes sclerodactylia or acrosclerosis.

Clinical Manifestations

Sclerodactylia characteristically begins between the ages of 30 and 50 and affects more women than men. The onset of systemic sclerosis is often a decade earlier. The patient has symptoms of digital ischemia over a prolonged period. At first cold numb fingers occur only under cold conditions, and attacks of Raynaud's phenomenon may occur; at this stage the condition may be labelled Raynaud's disease.

The true nature of the condition may be more quickly recognized if the possibility of scleroderma is considered. Sclerodermatous changes in the skin of the fingers result in loss of extensibility and mobility. At first the subcutaneous tissues may be swollen, giving the fingers a sausagelike appearance (Fig. 9-1). The matte surface of the skin becomes shiny, and the wrinkles of the

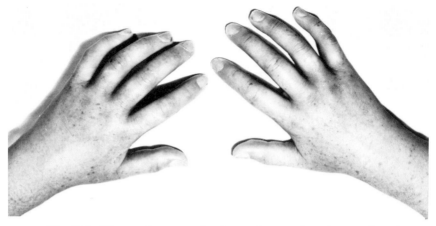

Fig. 9-1. Fingers in an early stage of acrosclerosis or sclerodactylia showing swollen sausagelike fingers and brown pigmentation
in the skin of the hands and forearms.

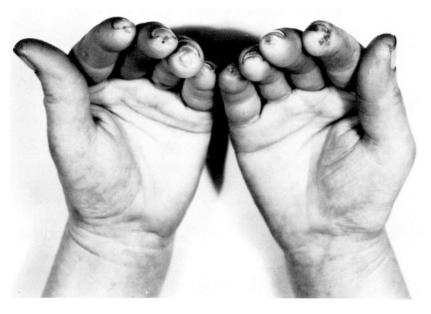

Fig. 9-2. Sclerodactylia in a later stage showing small necrotic
areas on the finger tips.

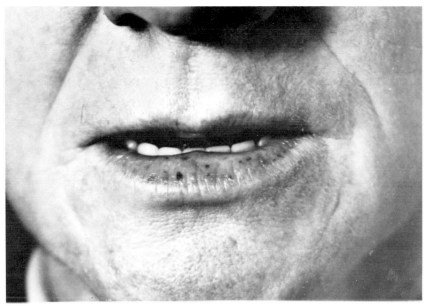

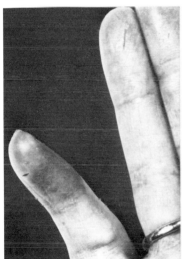
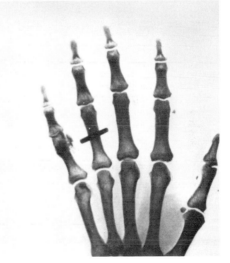

Fig. 9-3. (*a: Top*) Angiomata in lips and in skin of nose and cheeks of a female patient, age 45, with scleroderma. (*b: Bottom*) Calcification in soft tissues of hands and marked ischemia associated with the calcification in the little finger.

skin over the knuckles are smoothed out. As the skin loses its pliability it can no longer be pinched up from the dorsum of the fingers. With atrophy of the subcutaneous tissues the fingers become tapered and flexed and necrosis of their tips may occur (Fig. 9-2).

Toes are involved but seldom. The skin of the face is also liable to be affected. Tight skin is particularly noticeable over the forehead where the normal wrinkles are smoothed out and the skin can no longer be pinched up. The skin about the mouth appears to be atrophic with radial creases extending from the lips. The lips loose their suppleness so the mouth is restricted in the degree to which it can be opened. Ears may also be involved with thinning of the pinnae.

Disturbance of skin pigmentation is a feature of scleroderma: depigmented areas alternate with areas of increased pigmentation. This is particularly marked over the hands, but may also occur over the face and body. These pigment changes may occur in skin of normal mobility.

Small angiomata or telangiectases appear in the skin and mucous membranes (Fig. 9-3a). Deposits of calcium occur in the hands and sometimes in the pinnae of the ears; such deposits may precede other changes of scleroderma (Fig. 9-3b and 9-4). When it is realized that scleroderma, calcium deposition and telangiectases are all manifestations of the same disorder but seen to a different degree in different cases, it is clear that no useful purpose is served by the use of "roundsmanship" terms such as Thibierge-Weissenbach syndrome or the C.R.S.T. syndrome.

In the early stages of scleroderma the joints of the wrists and fingers are often painful, so that confusion with rheumatoid arthritis may occur. Arthritis may spread to elbows, knees and ankles, but the symptoms in the joints often diminish as other manifestations of scleroderma develop. In about a quarter of the cases permanent joint contractures and deformities develop, and rarely rheumatoid arthritis and scleroderma may coincide in the same patient. Synovial fibrosis occurs at the wrists and ankles, and tendon friction rubs may be heard. Difficulty in swallowing often occurs in the course of the disease.

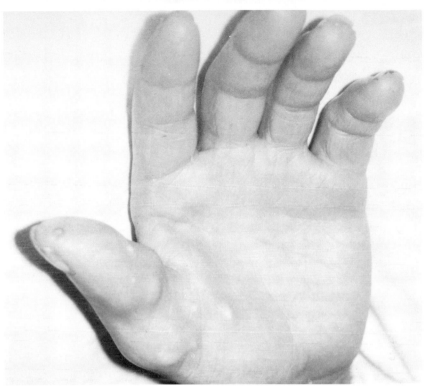

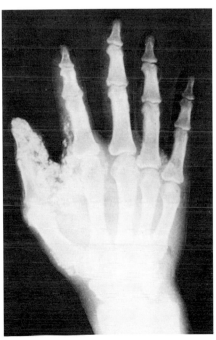

Fig. 9-4. Marked calcium deposits in the thenar space of the left hand of a man aged 32 years. His hand movements were impeded by the accumulation and were freed by its surgical removal. At the time of operation he was considered as a case of "calcinosis" and the only other sign of scleroderma were angiomata on the lips similar to those seen in Figure 9-3.

Late Manifestations

In many cases the painful digital lesions remain small, but in others a remorseless gnawing away of the fingers occurs (Fig. 9-5). A remarkable feature at this stage is the partial resorption of the ungual tuft of one or more fingers to complete dissolution of the terminal phalanges as well (Fig. 9-6). There is an imperfect correlation between the severity of the skin and vascular changes and the degree of bone resorption, and the phenomenon does not appear to be a simple consequence of digital ischemia.

Progressive pulmonary changes result in pulmonary hypertension and dyspnea. Sclerotic changes in the myocardium may show in the electrocardiogram. Chronic right heart failure is not common, for sudden death from a presumed myocardial infarct is a more frequent ending.

Dysphagia due to the lack of peristalsis in the esophagus is exacerbated by esophagitis, and serious weight loss and weakness result. Another cause of weight loss is involvement of the small intestine in the process with consequent malnutrition.

Investigations

The macroscopic changes in the skin are more characteristic than the microscopic changes, so confirmation of a clinical diagnosis by biopsy seems unnecessary. If the biopsy should be done through sclerodermatous skin, the healing of the incision is likely to be delayed, but if the biopsy is done through skin which is macroscopically normal, the pathologist may have to project to make his diagnosis.

Even if the patient has not complained of difficulty in swallowing, the demonstration of the weakening of propulsive forces in the lowest third of the esophagus is a most useful confirmatory sign. This can be done by radiographic examination which shows absence of peristalis in the affected region of the esophagus or preferably by recording of intraluminal pressures as the patient swallows.

Other laboratory findings tend to be confusing rather than helpful in the diagnosis of scleroderma. An increase in the

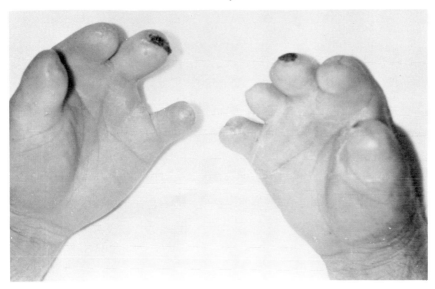

Fig. 9-5. Hands in late sclerodactylia.

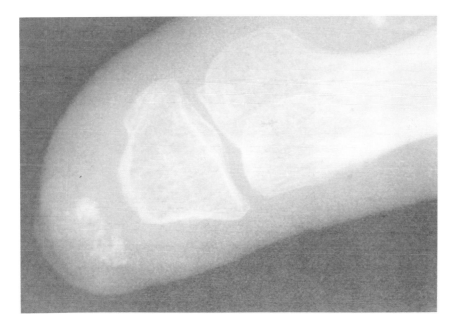

Fig. 9-6. Resorption of phalanges in sclerodactylia.

gamma globulins occurs in most cases, biological false positive tests for syphilis occur in a few cases, and occasionally an increased titer of antinuclear factor is found.

Treatment

The symptomatic treatment of sclerodactylia is described in Chapter 8. Sympathectomy is seldom of benefit, but considered amputation of affected digits or parts of digits may save the patient a great deal of pain.

In recent years no specific therapeutic agent for the sclerodermatous process has been advocated; but in the past relaxin, steroids, para-amino-benzoic acid, sodium versenate and antiserotonin agents have been advocated, tried, and found to be without effect on the sclerodermatous process. When ischemia is extensive and the possibility of obliteration of an artery exists (Fig. 9-7), arteriography should be carried out in the hope that an obstruction which is reparable by surgery may be found.

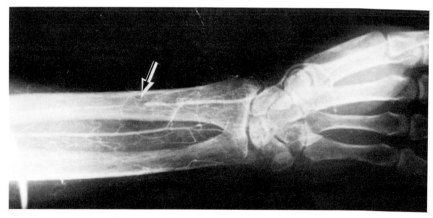

Fig. 9-7. A 39-year-old female whose condition had been diagnosed as scleroderma for 6 years developed gangrene of 3 fingers of the left hand. The arteriogram shows loss of the ulnar artery and block of a segment of the radial artery in the lower third of the forearm. Surgical repair of the radial artery by means of a vein graft resulted in increased blood flow to her hand. Local amputations of the affected digits healed successfully. (Report courtesy of Dr. Marvin Sachs and Dr. Clyde Barker.)

THROMBOANGIITIS OBLITERANS

Buerger's disease affects the arteries of the limbs distal to the elbows and below the knees. It occurs in young men and its clinical manifestations are quite distinct from those of arteriosclerosis obliterans (Table 9-1). In older patients both diseases may be

TABLE 9-1. ARTERIOSCLEROSIS OBLITERANS AND THROMBOANGIITIS OBLITERANS COMPARED

	A.S.O.	T.A.O.
Sex	⅔ male, ⅓ female	All male
Age of Onset	> 40	< 40
Cigarette Smoker	Often	Always
Response to Stopping Smoking	Little effect	Arrest of disease
Diabetes and/or Hyperlipidemia	Increased incidence	Normal incidence
Arteries Affected	Iliofemoral, coronary and cerebral	Radial, ulnar, peroneal and tibial, digital
Superficial Phlebitis	Rare	Frequent

present. The relationship between cigarette smoking and Buerger's disease is a very close one: if a patient stops smoking his disease is arrested, if he takes up smoking again the disease progresses. For unknown reasons the disease has become quite rare during the past quarter century.

The histological appearance of vessels affected by thromboangiitis obliterans differs from that of arteriosclerotic vessels by the appearance of recanalizing thrombus in the lumina of the vessels, by the well preserved medial coats, and by the invasion of media and adventitia by lymphocytes and fibroblasts. However, in old lesions obtained from amputated limbs these distinctions may be slight. Angiography shows attenuated lumina of the tibial, radial, and ulnar arteries. The affected segments are long, and many helical collateral channels open up around the involved arteries. The appearance is characteristic (Fig. 9-8).

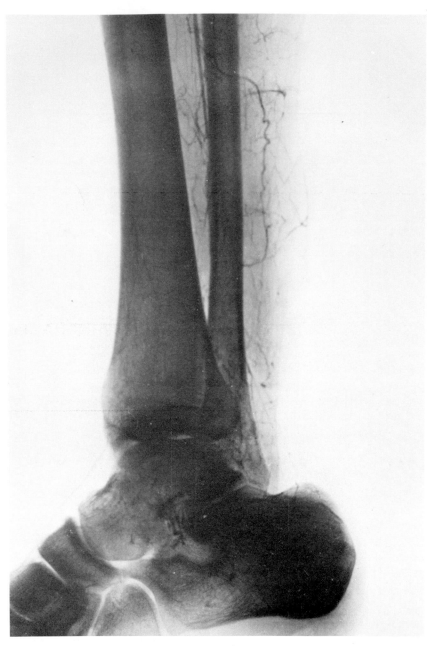
Fig. 9-8. Arteriogram of patient with thromboangiitis obliterans showing distal block of tibial and peroneal arteries and proliferation of collateral circulation in calf.

Clinical Manifestations

Persistent pain in a cyanosed and cold toe is often the earliest symptom (Fig. 9-9), though occasionally a finger may first give rise to symptoms. Intermittent claudication is the first complaint of some patients, and when, as often happens in many of these cases, the pain occurs in the arch of the foot, it may be mistaken for an orthopedic difficulty. Written accounts stress superficial phlebitis as an early sign, though the minority of cases demonstrate it. However, when superficial phlebitis occurs in a young man, particular attention should be paid to the state of his arterial circulation.

Even at this stage of the earliest symptoms the arteries of the calf or forearm are already extensively affected. If symptoms occur in the hands it is unusual for either radial or ulnar artery to be palpable, or if in the foot, for dorsalis pedis or posterior tibial pulse to be felt. To quote Sir Thomas Lewis, "There is no other disease which brings such universal ruin to the large and small arteries of a limb; and there is none in which the extent of vascular obliteration is so disproportionate to the symptoms."

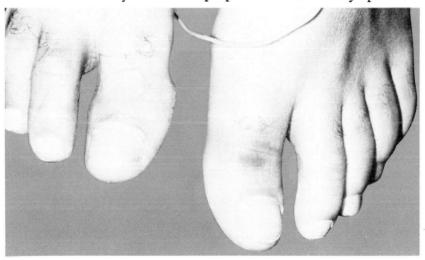

Fig. 9-9. Persistent cyanosis and coldness of left great toe in early thromboangiitis obliterans.

This is due to the fact that development of collateral arterial channels almost keeps pace with the obliteration of the regular arteries so that, though the main arteries are blocked, metabolic needs are almost served by the collateral circulation. It is necessary to qualify the fine sweep of Sir Thomas' statement, for though arteries distal to the elbows and knees are extensively obliterated, the upper brachial and femoral arteries are rarely diseased, unless by an acute thrombosis within them as a result of the diminution of flow through them. Visceral arteries such as the coronary and cerebral are never, or almost never, involved. The reports of involvement of arteries other than those distal to the elbow and knee should be accepted only with reserve. In particular it must be recognized that thromboangiitis at 35 years of age affords no protection from atherosclerosis obliterans 10 or 15 years later and that when patients with thromboangiitis live longer, the combined effects of the two diseases are seen more often.

Treatment

Unless the patient stops smoking, treatment is of little avail. Because the main incidence of the disease is on the distal arteries of the legs rather than on the proximal arteries, lumbar sympathectomy is often of value in so improving the circulation that healing of lesions occurs. Amputation frequently has to be done, but fortunately the local amputation of a digit will usually heal satisfactorily. No special study of the effect of sympatheticolytic drugs appears to have been carried out in Buerger's disease, but because of the usefulness of sympathectomy it is possible that they may be of help.

CRANIAL ARTERITIS AND POLYMYALGIA RHEUMATICA

The names temporal arteritis, senile arteritis, giant cell arteritis and Horton's arteritis, and also polymyalgia arteritica and polymyalgia rheumatica all refer to an arterial disease of the elderly which is increasing in frequency. The arteritis occurs mostly in patients over 60 years of age and predominantly affects the carotids and their branches. The temporal arteries as they run in the scalp are particularly affected causing severe headache with local tenderness, redness, and swelling amounting on occasion to actual gangrene. It has been recognized that in many cases the acute temporal arteritis is preceded by polymyalgia rheumatica.

The latter condition is defined as a protracted disease of the elderly characterized by proximal pain and stiffness, general illness, mild anemia, and a raised sedimentation rate. A typical case history would be of general malaise with "rheumatic" pains which are felt proximally, that is around the shoulders, neck, spine, hips and thighs. Initially they may be in one region only, but as time goes on they tend to affect both sides equally. The pains and stiffness are felt particularly in the morning and may make getting out of bed an agonizing experience. The joints are not swollen. At this stage a sedimentation rate of over 35 mm./hour should lead to investigation to eliminate myeloma, "collagen diseases," carcinoma, leukemia and other diseases. When such serious possibilities have been eliminated a trial of steroid treatment should be made, and if a rapid response occurs it is reasonable to make a diagnosis of "polymyalgia rheumatica." If at this stage the disease is not recognized and treated, temporal arteritis is liable to ensue in weeks, months, or years. In the quiet interim, biopsy of the temporal artery or other affected cranial artery may show large celled arteritis in about one third of the patients (St. J. Dixon), and pulsation in the temporal arteries may disappear at any time.

The acute attack of arteritis begins with severe frontal and temporal headaches, unilateral at first and then bilateral. The temporal artery is swollen and tender; pulsations increase at first and decrease later, when the artery may be felt as a cord. Ophthalmoscopic examination may show an optic neuritis. Muscles in the area of supply of the temporal artery may be affected by intermittent claudication so that the patient cannot finish a meal of solid food. Neurological manifestations such as vertigo, disorientation, delirium, and diplopia, and visual disturbances such as diminished vision and flashes of light may occur. These symptoms suggest cerebral involvement.

The diagnosis is clinched when a biopsy of the temporal artery shows the typical giant celled arteritis; this procedure may incidentally relieve the symptoms. However, treatment should not wait for this confirmation because the danger of sudden blindness is a real one. Steroid treatment should be begun on suspicion and continued in doses sufficient to suppress the sedimentation rate to below 20 mm./hour in men and 30 mm./hour in women. Continuation of the treatment may be required for years.

PERIARTERITIS NODOSA

In 1866 Kussmaul and Maier described gross and microscopic pathological specimens which showed focal inflammation of small and medium sized arteries. Many of the lesions were found in renal tissue and had come from cases of "Bright's Disease" by which term albuminuria, hypertension, and renal failure were implied. After 40 years a similar condition was described in the English language and in this description emphasis was placed on the many tissues and vessels which might be affected so that the alternate name, polyarteritis, was suggested. Since then numerous cases with focal inflammatory lesions of medium sized and small arteries have been described, and to peri- and poly- the name panarteritis has been added. There is no single criterion by which the clinical entity of periarteritis may be recognized, but the category is a useful one in practice, even if several as yet undifferentiated disease entities may prove to have been included under this term. In 1957 Rose and Spencer reviewed 104 cases of disseminated arteritis which had been recorded as periarteritis nodosa. They separated them into two categories according to the presence or absence of pulmonary artery involvement. In the absence of pulmonary involvement the criteria for diagnosis of periarteritis were usually complied with, but when pulmonary arteries were affected, it seemed likely that allergic angiitis, with or without granulomatosis, would have been a more correct nomenclature. From this study it would seem that pulmonary arteries are seldom involved in periarteritis nodosa, though bronchial arteries often are.

Though periarteritis nodosa is still an uncommon disease, an apparent increase in its incidence and the incidence of its variants has occurred in the last 30 years. The impression that periarteritis was more frequently diagnosed after sulfonamide had come into general use and the experimental demonstration by Rich and Gregory that a periarteritis could be a manifestation of hypersensitivity to sulfonamides implicated immunologic mechanisms in its pathogenesis. It does have clinical features similar to those of other immunological disorders such as systemic lupus erythematosus, and in some patients the disease appears to have been provoked by a sensitivity reaction to serum, or drugs such as penicillin, thiouracil, or sulfonamide.

Classically periarteritis affects large muscular arterioles near bifurcations or at the hilar regions of viscera, although small arterioles may also be involved. The pulmonary circulation and spleen are usually spared. In contrast, hypersensitivity vasculitis involves small arteries, capillaries and venules and frequently affects the lungs and spleen. No diagnostic test such as the demonstration of antinuclear factor in systemic lupus erythematosus has been discovered for periarteritis.

The type of illness that is diagnosed as periarteritis nodosa is one occurring between the ages of twenty and fifty, though occasionally cases may be recognized in infancy or in old age. Males are more commonly affected than females, but the reported ratio of 3 or 4 males to 1 female is not particularly helpful in differential diagnosis. Suspicion of the disease is likely to be aroused by such obscure indications as nonspecific fever, progressive decline in general health with evidence of involvement of several organs and tissues in particular the kidneys, gastrointestinal tract, and peripheral arteries and nerves. Laboratory studies may show a rapid sedimentation rate, leukocytosis with or without eosinophilia. Focal arterial inflammation in biopsy specimens is to be looked, for but it is not clear which tissue should be used for this biopsy; the kidney is most often advised but other authors consider biopsy of the liver or testes as being more informative. Most would not encourage random biopsy of muscle. A positive result on biopsy provides the best diagnostic evidence of the disease, though a negative result does not exclude the diagnosis. A recent advance in the diagnosis of periarteritis has been the use of renal angiography. By this technique, typically segmental lesions of the arteries with aneurysmal formation may be seen in the distal segmental, interlobar, and possibly the arcuate arteries. The arteriographic changes selected from these studies for publication are striking and would appear to correlate well with the underlying histopathologic changes. When present they appear to be a strong diagnostic finding, though at this time there has not been sufficient experience of the investigation to indicate what is the incidence of such arteriographic changes in periarteritis nodosa, nor whether similar changes may be found in other vascular diseases such as systemic lupus erythematosus, gram negative septicemia, malignant hypertension, or the vasculitis associated with rheumatoid disease.

Periarteritis nodosa is not a uniformly fatal disease, and its progression is as variable as its other features; its course may run from a few weeks to many months, or even years. Periods of remission and relapse occur, and some patients recover entirely from the disease.

Manifestations in the Extremities

In the description of scleroderma it was stated that two forms of the disease may be distinguished: one in which the brunt is on the viscera (systemic sclerosis), the other in which digital ischemia is the major manifestation (sclerodactylia). No such clear distinction can be made in the case of periarteritis nodosa, but in a description of peripheral arterial disease it is of value to emphasize manifestations of the disease in the extremities rather than those in the viscera. When the distinction between predominantly systemic and predominantly peripheral periarteritis nodosa can be made, it is a useful one for when the disease affects predominantly the peripheral arteries the chances of recovery from it appear to be greater.

Subcutaneous aneurysmal nodules would be a finding most in favor of periarteritis nodosa. In the earlier recorded cases such nodules were found on digital arteries and even on arteries as large as the ulnar, and it was this finding which was likely to prompt the diagnosis. At the present time these nodules are found in a minority of cases, and it is other manifestations which lead to the diagnosis.

A peripheral manifestation more frequently found is that of ischemic changes and even gangrene of the fingers and toes. In the early stages the digits show persistent ischemia with pallor and cyanosis, and they are usually painful (Fig. 8-4). The condition often progresses to gangrene, though pulsation in the named arteries and sometimes even in the digital arteries persists. The gross changes resemble those found in rheumatoid arthritis or systemic lupus erythematosus. They differ from embolic manifestations in that they do not appear suddenly but take hours or days to develop; though localized they are not so punctate as the lesions caused by small emboli, and they may, often do, occur in fingers and toes simultaneously. Associated with these acral changes there is often evidence of restricted cutaneous circulation to more proximal parts of limb in the form of livedo reticularis, petechiae, ecchymoses, purpura, and urticaria.

Nonspecific myalgias and arthralgias occur in about half the cases, and joint swelling and atrophy of the muscles from focal necrosis and disuse may follow.

Symptoms referable to peripheral nerves are common, and apparently are due to ischemia caused by involvement of the vasa nervorum. These occur in about half the cases. In one quarter of cases, such peripheral neuritis is the presenting feature of the disease. The initial symptoms of pain, paresthesias and weakness occur rather more commonly in the lower extremities than the upper, though with progress of the disease both lower and upper extremities tend to be involved. Motor changes are more prominent than sensory, though usually both are present. Patients with involvement of peripheral nerves subdivide into two approximately equal categories. One half manifest the characteristic mononeuritis multiplex; finding of involvement of sensory and motor functions of several nerve trunks in any obscure illness is practically diagnostic of periarteritis nodosa. In the other half of patients with involvement of peripheral nerves the pattern is that of a symmetrical multiple neuritis which on clinical examination is in no way different from that encountered in toxic or infectious polyneuritis.

Which ever manifestations occur in the limbs, the recognition of the disease usually arises from detection of evidence of systemic involvement. Most often this is of renal changes with hypertension, though central nervous involvement is not uncommon, or involvement of any portion of the G.I. tract, liver, gall bladder, or pancreas.

Treatment

When the diagnosis of periarteritis nodosa is reasonably sure, vigorous treatment with adrenal corticosteroids is required to control symptoms and attempt to arrest the progress of the disease. Prednisone is begun at a dose of 60 mg. daily and occasionally an even higher dose may be required. In favorable cases general symptomatic improvement, regression of lesions, and a return of the sedimentation rate to normal may be hoped for. The medication is continued in high doses for weeks or months until evidence of regression is obtained when the dose is tapered. Tapering implies reduction of the daily dose to levels of 20 to 30 mg. daily with subsequent reduction by 5 mg. monthly or at longer intervals to avoid exacerbation of the disease. Sometimes the medication may be stopped, though in most cases prolonged maintenance therapy is required. In other less favorable cases a worsening of the condition occurs with steroid therapy, but even in these cases a prolonged trial of steroid therapy should be maintained for eventually some degree of remission may occur. In Fronert and Sheps' long term follow-up study of 130 patients with histological evidence of PAN, the 5-year survival was 48 per cent for patients treated with adrenal corticosteroids and 13 per cent for patients not so treated. Patients with hypertension and renal disease at the outset of treatment did not respond well, whereas pulmonary involvement did not greatly influence the course of the disease. The majority of patients required continuing steroid treatment to suppress symptoms or to prevent exacerbations.

General principles of treatment for the peripheral vascular phenomena must be followed. Surgical amputation of affected digits is not recommended because healing of the amputation site is slow.

PULSELESS DISEASE, TAKAYASU'S DISEASE, OR AORTIC ARCH SYNDROME

Nomenclature

In May 1905 Takayasu described a female patient who had complained of dimness of vision for 8 months. The remarkable finding in her was a wreath of anastomotic vessels surrounding the optic disc at a distance of 2 to 3 mm., and surrounding this another circle of anastomoses. She subsequently developed cataracts and a retinal detachment. In the discussion which followed Onishi described a similar case but with the added findings that her arms were cold and that her radial pulses could not be felt. Since then reports, mostly from Japan, have described what appears to be a specific disease affecting primarily the subclavian and carotid arteries. Only rarely is a typical case reported from North America or Europe.

As the condition has been defined it consists of blockage of the carotid and subclavian arteries at their origin from the arch of the aorta and for some distance along their length. Blockage of the subclavian arteries results in loss of pulsation in the upper extremities which gives rise to the name of pulseless disease. Pulses persist in the lower extremities because the lumen of the aorta is free, and for this reason the condition is sometimes referred to as reversed coarctation. The condition is so rare outside Japan and neighboring countries that it is unlikely that a physician in this country will ever see a case, but it is described here as an example of a specific form of arterial disease.

Definition

The use of angiography has resulted in definite information on the location and extent of arterial involvement in Takayasu's syndrome. The observations of Sano et al. in a series of 31 cases show a remarkable pattern of involvement. There was a preponderance of arterial occlusion of the left side, with the left subclavian artery being most frequently affected and the right vertebral artery, least. One half of the cases had bilateral carotid artery occlusion; among those with unilateral occlusions, 12 occurred on the left side and only four on the right. Bilateral subclavian occlusion occurred in 22 cases, but in all 31 the left subclavian artery was narrowed. The left vertebral artery was narrowed in 12, but most remarkably, in no case was the right vertebral artery narrowed. Development of collateral circulation in the thyroid and substernal arterial anastomoses was a feature of the angiograms. Though left subclavian occlusion occurred in all 31 cases and right vertebral occlusion in none, the subclavian steal phenomenon was seen in only eight cases, for the subclavian occlusion was usually distal to the origin of the vertebral artery.

The ascending aorta was not affected, but the descending aorta was narrowed in four cases just distal to the left subclavian and in another three, at the level of the renal arteries. It has been stated elsewhere that occlusion of the aorta and renal arteries occurs predominantly in young people and is associated with a poor prognosis, arterial hypertension being almost invariably associated.

Reports on narrowing of the coronary arteries have been less precise but may be expected to be more defined with the increasing use of coronary angiography. In the patient I observed personally the angiographic report was of probable narrowing of the right coronary artery, though she had no symptoms of angina, and the electrocardiogram showed only nonspecific ST depressions.

In the past decade obliteration of the pulmonary arteries has been reported fairly frequently as a feature of the disease. Incompetence of the aortic valve is also being more frequently recognized.

Female patients preponderate, and only rarely is the authentic disease seen in a male. In the majority of cases the disorder starts around the age of 20, but it may appear as early as 8 years, and cases first diagnosed after the age of 40 have been reported.

Histological examination of the affected vessels shows them to be obliterated by a chronic inflammatory process, with infiltration of the wall with round cells and giant cells. Calcification is rare and occurs only in older patients.

Etiology

When the disease was first described an association with tuberculous infection was suggested. Later, because of confusion with syphilitic aortitis and the occurrence of false biological positive serological reaction, syphilis was implicated. More recently it has been pointed out that the disease affects arteries known to have a large component of elastic tissue in their walls and seems to spare arteries with preponderantly muscular walls. Sano has described the finding of autoantibodies against the aortic wall, presumably against the elastic component.

Symptoms

The disease commonly starts with an acute febrile illness with nasopharyngeal and pulmonary infections. Erythema nodosum and arthralgias sometimes occur during the acute phase. Pleuritis, pleural effusion and pericarditis may also occur. Pulses are usually still present at this stage.

A slow progression of arterial obstruction with simultaneous development of collateral circulation follows the acute phase. The symptoms can be divided into cerebral: giddiness, faintness, and syncope, brachial: coldness, paresthesias, and easy fatigue of the arms, and ophthalmic: diminished visual acuity.

The cerebral symptoms appear to be due to cerebral ischemia, but cerebrovascular accidents are uncommon. This may be attributable to adequate collateral circulation because the branches of the circle of Willis are not affected, and collateral circulation between the transcervical arteries is good. It also seems that the arterial disease does not give rise to emboli, as does atherosclerosis.

In some cases intermittent claudication of the muscles used in mastication has been described. The brachial symptoms tend to be dismissed as "not true intermittent claudication," but the aching and fatigue of the arms is a very troublesome complaint which interferes with such everyday occupations as dressing one's hair. Rather unexpectedly, Raynaud's phenomenon is an unusual complaint, though coldness of the hands is complained of.

Transient visual disturbances are reported in 70 per cent of the cases, and cataracts develop in 45 per cent. In the majority of cases ophthalmic symptoms are less troublesome than the cerebral or the brachial.

Signs

The outstanding sign of pulseless disease is diminished brachial pulsations resulting in absence of the radial pulse and difficulty in measuring the brachial arterial pressure. Somewhat facetiously, McKusick has suggested that the condition is more frequently recognized if the system of medicine used is based on Chinese medical techniques. This is because the Chinese way of medicine emphasizes the importance of careful bilateral examination of the radial pulse.

Common findings are persistent tachycardia and hypertension, the latter being measured in the lower extremities. Both have been attributed to lowered pressure in the carotid sinus, though hypertension is often related to renal artery involvement.

Loss of hair and atrophy of the facial muscles has been attributed to the ischemia.

The eyes may show some degree of enophthalmos with atropy of the iris and uveal tract as well as the cataracts and retinal changes originally described. Though the retinal manifestations were what first called Takayasu's attention to the disease, it is now recognized that the anastomoses seen round the optic discs are indicative of lowered retinal arterial pressure rather than being specific to the disease.

Cardiac hypertrophy, attributable to hypertension or aortic regurgitation, is often found. The aortic diastolic murmur must be carefully listened for.

Stenosis of the subclavian artery, particularly on the left, gives rise to a continuous murmur, sometimes described as a machinery murmur. The genesis of the diastolic component has been attributed to a very low pressure distal to the stenosis, but when aortic regurgitation is present the murmur may be a truly to and fro murmur due to the reversal of blood flow in the aortic root during diastole. Whatever its cause, the continuous murmur in this site may be mistaken for that of a patent ductus arteriosus.

Development of collateral circulation in the upper thoracic region may result in paravertebral systolic murmurs, as in coarctation of the aorta, though the flow within the vessels is in the opposite direction. With the background of this pandemonium of thoracic murmurs it is not surprising that the quiet murmur of pulmonary artery stenosis has not been recognized.

Upper abdominal murmurs may arise when there is involvement of the aorta and renal arteries. In the case I examined the femoral pulses were forcible, and pistol shot sounds were heard over them.

Laboratory Findings

There is often a mild anemia. An elevated sedimentation rate is almost invariably found, with an elevation of the globulin, particularly the gamma fraction. The C reactive proteins are also often increased. Positive LE preps, latex fixation, antithyroid autoantibodies, false biologically positive test for syphilis, and polyarteritis nodosa-like biopsies have all been reported in occasional cases. Changes in lipoproteins are not to be expected.

Angiography of the vessels of the aortic arch shows the degree of involvement of the arteries. Lung scans will indicate whether pulmonary arteries are involved, and pulmonary and coronary angiography are indicated in the investigation of future cases.

Diagnosis

Diagnosis of the disease in the initial febrile state "pulseless disease with pulses" is probably not possible under ordinary circumstances. Arteries are said to be sensitive to pressure in these early stages, but this sign is not likely to be sought, and even if found, not likely to be considered diagnostic.

As the disease develops it might be thought that it could be confused with polymyalgia rheumatica and giant cell arteritis, but the young age of the patients with pulseless disease is very much against the diagnosis of these conditions. When the striking angiographic findings are associated with stenosis of the pulmonary arteries and aortic regurgitation in a young female there would seem to be little doubt of the diagnosis.

Most of the cases recognized in Europe and North America have been in females over the age of 35, and the distinction between unusual atheroma and pulseless disease in them may be very difficult to make. There are angiographic points of distinction between atheromatous disease and pulseless disease. One is that in atheroma the carotid bifurcations and the first part of the subclavian arteries are often affected, whereas they seldom are in pulseless disease. Another is that the narrowing caused by pulseless disease appears as a smooth segmental narrowing 3 to 5 cm. long, rather than as the irregular encroachment of atheroma into the lumen of the artery.

For 10 years we have been caring for a woman of 49 who has stenosis of subclavian and carotid arteries with consequent manifestations of pulseless disease. She told me that her condition had been so diagnosed by a physician who has written on the disease and who might well be termed an authority. However, in spite of the absence of pulses in her arms the following points are more in favor of her disease being atherosclerosis than pulseless disease. (1) The trouble began with aortoiliac obstruction which has not been described as an area of obstruction in the classic cases of the disease; (2) the angiographic appearance of the carotid arteries resembled atheroma rather than pulseless disease; (3) she derived decided benefit from endoarterectomy and bypass procedures; and (4) microscopic examination of the diseased artery resected during arterial reconstruction did not show any inflammatory cells.

Treatment and Prognosis

Steroid treatment has been claimed to be beneficial, but the effects appear to be nonspecific and to have little or no effect on the prolonged course of the disease. Chloroquine and antimetabolites have been used without notable success. By the time arterial surgery is considered, the disease is usually extensive so that surgical repair presents considerable technical difficulties. There are few reports of successful carotid arterial surgery for this condition in the literature.

Against this depressing account of the effects of treatment can be placed the relatively good prognosis indicated by a follow-up of cases. In a series of 20 patients observed for up to 20 years only 4 deaths occurred, 3 due to left heart failure and one of a probable myocardial infarct. As noted above, there were no cerebrovascular incidents.

SECONDARY VASCULAR DISEASES

SYSTEMIC LUPUS ERYTHEMATOSUS

SLE is a multisystem disorder. Lesions may develop in skin, kidney, heart, central nervous system, synovial and serous membranes, and in the G.I. tract and liver, but the involvement of one organ may overshadow that of others for long periods. It has been said that SLE has supplanted syphilis as the "great imitator," not merely because of the occurrence of false positive serological tests for syphilis during the course of the disease but because any organ may be affected and many symptom complexes arise.

It has been customary to include SLE in accounts of vascular disease, and so it is included here. However, as the account shows, vascular manifestations (vasculitis) are probably secondary to the immunologic features. Therefore this disease has been placed in this section of vascular complications of general disease.

Immunologic Features

Many of the immunological abnormalities which have been described in SLE are nonspecific in that they may be associated with a wide variety of other diseases. Over the years the search for an abnormality specific to the condition has narrowed and at the present time the activity in the serum of antibodies against native or double-stranded DNA may prove to be a specific indication of the activity of the disorder.

In about one half of cases of SLE serum globulin concentrations are found in excess of 4.10 g. per 100 ml., but the globulins are heterogeneous (γ, β_2, and α) rather than of a specific type. Antibodies to red cells (Coombs' test) are occasionally present and associated with a hemolytic anemia. The occasional appearance of a bleeding diathesis may be linked to a thrombocytopenic purpura or the presence of antibodies to blood clotting factors in the serum. An antibody which causes false positive tests for syphilis may be present for months or years before overt manifestations of SLE occur. This test forms a useful step in making a diagnosis.

More directly related to diagnosis of the disease was the discovery in 1948 of the LE phenomenon which many patients with SLE will develop sometime during their illness, though a negative finding does not exclude the disease. Since introduction of the LE test, a variety of circulating antibodies directed against various components of the cell nucleus have been described. The most widely used of these is a test for antinuclear factor using immunofluorescence. There is a subjective element in the interpretation of titers of ANF to account for the conditions under which the test was performed. Nevertheless this test is likely to be positive when SLE is active, and serial determinations may prove of value in the management of a patient's illness.

More recently, tests for antinuclear factors appear to have been made more specific by elaboration of methods to detect circulating antibodies to native or double-stranded DNA. The presence of these antibodies in the circulating blood has been considered to indicate an immulogic hyperreactivity (humoral) characteristic of patients with SLE. In one series, high titers of anti-DNA activity were found in patients in whom the disease was considered to be an active disease. Of particular diagnostic import in these observations was that the serum of patients with a variety of diseases other than SLE which had positive ANF or LE cell tests, did not show activity of DNA antibodies. Also, the serum of patients with drug-induced lupus with positive ANF and/or positive LE cell tests did not show anti-DNA activity. If such remarkable specificity of the test is still found on wider usage it will be clear that a useful diagnostic test has been found, the genesis of SLE has been made clearer, and greater effort can be directed to the question of how and why circulating antibodies to DNA arise in this condition. Already the observations have further provided a stimulus to investigate the possibility that viral infections may release DNA into the circulation, and from this cause antibodies to it arise.

With the greater importance of immunological factors in the causation of SLE vascular phenomena are less etiologically significant, though they may not be overlooked.

Vascular Manifestations

Raynaud's phenomenon is often cited as a presenting sign of SLE. The diagnostic value of this observation is hard to assess because, as described in Chapter 8, the term Raynaud's phenomenon is used loosely, and the idiopathic form of Raynaud's phenomenon is not uncommon in females at the age when they are liable to develop the more unusual systemic lupus erythematosus. More characteristic of SLE is the appearance of evanescent erythematous nodules and small punctate ulcerative lesions on the fingers and palms which sometimes progress to digital gangrene. Similar ulcerations may be found on mucous membranes. These lesions are more indicative of SLE than the more frequently encountered Raynaud's phenomenon; they may indicate an underlying vasculitis, but perhaps they are more likely to be the result of cutaneous immunological reactions.

The erythematous, scaling, dislike plaques characteristic of discoid lupus erythematosus also occur in SLE, but they appear to be more an inflammatory lesion than one of primary vasculitis, particularly since they are exacerbated by exposure to ultraviolet radiation.

Another lesion occurring in SLE which has been attributed to "vasculitis" is aseptic necrosis of bone. Necrosis of bone usually requires a blood supply adequate for the metabolism of osteoclasts and the removal of calcium, so a vasculitis with restricted blood supply would be an unlikely explanation of this phenomenon. A more likely process would seem to be an inflammatory mechanism, and in none of the reported cases has a primary impairment of blood supply by vasculitis been demonstrated. The relationship of aseptic necrosis to steroid therapy is uncertain, for osseous necrosis of the type called aseptic necrosis may occur in conditions other than SLE which have not been treated with steroids. Aseptic necrosis has, moreover, been reported in patients with SLE who were not receiving steroids at the onset of symptoms.

Venous thrombosis occurs more frequently in SLE than would be expected by chance, and we have seen one patient who developed venous gangrene (phlegmasia cerulea dolens) during the course of the disease.

In summary, the evidence that SLE is the cause of "vasculitis" and is responsible for symptoms of the peripheral vascular system is unconvincing, and to press the assertion adds to the confusion inherent in the term collagen vascular disease.

SYSTEMIC "ALLERGIC" VASCULITIS (INCLUDING RHEUMATOID ARTHRITIS)

The term vasculitis implies an inflammatory reaction of small arteries and veins and the capillaries between them. The causes of this reaction are many, for it would seem that the microvasculature has but one response to a wide series of noxious agents. Some of these agents such as bacterial, viral, and heterologous serum antigens with their reactive antibodies are recognizable, as are pharmacologic agents such as penicillin, sulfonamide and chloramphenicol. Less defined at present are the agents responsible for the vasculitis associated with rheumatoid arthritis, but it would seem that these are auto-antibodies. Still unrecognized are the agents responsible for Wegener's granulomatosis and erythema nodosum. In contrast to systemic lupus erythematosus, vasculitis affects males almost as often as females, and older rather than younger people.

Some conditions render a person more disposed to the development of vasculitis. A history of allergic diseases such as infantile eczema, bronchial asthma, hay fever and urticaria are such manifestations. Chronic leukemia and low grade lymphoma also appear to render a person more prone to the development of vasculitis. Whether rheumatoid arthritis and associated steroid therapy are a causative or exacerbating factor for vasculitis is not clear.

In most forms of vasculitis the cause appears to be the attachment of molecular complexes formed by the union of antigen and antibody onto the endothelial cells of small blood vessels where they give rise to an inflammatory reaction. By means of fluorescent techniques such complexes have been seen in apposition with the endothelial cells. This process may occur widely over the circulation or be confined to vessels of a particular region, the skin and kidney in particular. Because this process may affect any organ, a variety of syndromes result from it, and to describe them all is not within the compass of this work. The syndromes which may be included under the category of systemic allergic vasculitis are: rheumatoid arteritis, Wegener's granulomatosis, serum sickness, vascular drug reactions, vascular (anaphylactoid) purpura, microscopic polyarteritis, allergic granulomatosis, hypersensitivity angiitis, "allergic" vasculitis (angiitis), and arteriolitis "allergica" cutis.

Rheumatoid Arteritis

The most frequently encountered vasculitis encountered by the physician interested in vascular diseases is that associated with rheumatoid arthritis. This vasculitis has been reported to occur more frequently with the development of subcutaneous nodules, it is also believed that it occurs more frequently since the introduction of steroid therapy.

An early manifestation of vasculitis in rheumatoid arthritis is the appearance of punctate vascular lesions in the pads of the toes and fingers, though it may also first manifest itself by the acute onset of a peroneal palsy. The digital lesions may recur intermittently over many years, or they may progress rapidly to gangrene of the digit. The skin of the patient with rheumatoid arthritis is thin and delicate and is more likely to be so if he has been on steroid therapy so that coalescence of the punctate lesions appears to occur easily and very painful necrosis of the fingers to result.

The relationship of this form of vasculitis to steroid therapy is not clear. It is certain that the majority of patients with rheumatoid arthritis who develop vasculitis have been treated with steroids, and the disease appears to have become more common since the introduction of steroid therapy. However, rheumatoid arteritis was described before the introduction of steroid therapy, and patients with other diseases, such as bronchial asthma, treated with steroids do not appear to be so prone to the development of vasculitis. If arteritis is precipitated by steroid therapy it is paradoxical that there is general agreement that at least a temporary increase in steroid dosage is required for its treatment. The use of antimetabolic drugs to permit early tapering of the steroid dosage may be of some value, but it has not yet come into general use.

The occurrence of vasculitis in the digits of patients with rheumatoid arthritis prompted an angiographic study of the digital arteries in this condition. It was found that patients with rheumatoid arthritis are liable to intimal thickening and thrombosis of the digital arteries. Clinical evidence of this arterial narrowing may or may not be present during life, moreover it is not invariable even in the presence of long-standing and severe seropositive rheumatoid disease. One patient with widespread necrotising vasculitis supervening on rheumatoid disease showed only simple intimal thickening in the digital arteries. The relationship between these two types of vascular lesion in rheumatoid arthritis is not clear, but it would seem that if narrowing of the digital arteries has occurred the effects of vasculitis in the smaller vessels would be felt more severely.

Laboratory Abnormalities. Leukocytosis, if it occurs in association with vasculitis, is of moderate degree (10 to 20,000). Eosinophilia is uncommon in spite of the allergic background. Elevation of the blood sedimentation rate is by far the most common hematologic abnormality; this is associated with an elevation of serum globulins.

Lupus erythematosus cells are not found, and antinuclear serum tests are negative. In cases of rheumatoid angiitis, high titers of rheumatoid factor are common. Biopsy of affected tissues shows inflammatory reaction bordering on the microvasculature.

POLYCYTHEMIA VERA AND THROMBOCYTHEMIA

In one series of 250 patients with polycythemia vera, two thirds had at least one thrombotic complication, either arterial or venous, during their course, and in 40 per cent death was attributable directly to thrombosis. Patients with polycythemia secondary to an hypoxic condition also have an increased danger of arterial and venous thromboses. The cause of this increased tendency to thrombosis has not progressed beyond the observation of Osler that the blood in this disease is "thick and sticky." If atherosclerotic plaques restrict the free flow of blood in the arteries, the degree of polycythemia may determine whether or not ischemic manifestations develop. Raynaud's phenomenon is relatively infrequent in polycythemia vera, but complaints of burning pain in the extremities (erythermalgia) are frequently heard.

Thrombotic incidents are reduced if the red cell mass and the hematocrit can be reduced to normal. This is routinely accomplished by venesection. The use of anticoagulants carries some risk because of the hemorrhagic tendency which frequently exists in these patients, but cautious use of heparin is permissible whilst the hematocrit is being brought under control.

Of particular interest are patients with little or no elevation of red cell count but a two- or threefold elevation of the platelet count. These patients appear to be as prone to thrombosis as those with elevated red cell counts, and the cause of their thrombotic tendency may not be recognized unless a platelet count is specified. For the patient whose platelet count rises dangerously following phlebotomy, myelosuppression with radioactive phosphorus is the preferred treatment. In a recently reported case it was found that the platelets were functionally abnormal in that they aggregated spontaneously in platelet-rich plasma. The spontaneous aggregation could be inhibited by aminophenazone or aspirin, and on treatment with these agents the patient remained free, not only of attacks of venous thrombosis, but also of attacks of erythermalgia in toes and fingers. Coumarin treatment had no apparent effect on the effects of the platelet aggregation.

POST-TRAUMATIC REFLEX SYMPATHETIC DYSTROPHY

In 1864 Silas Weir Mitchell, G. R. Moorhouse, and W. W. Keen (the last named, a renowned surgeon, many years later was called in to assist in the secret operation on the sarcomatous upper jaw of President Cleveland) described a complication of gun shot wounds in Civil War soldiers. It was a burning pain (causalgia) following injury, but not severance, of a peripheral nerve. Since that time it has been observed that the same condition may follow trauma to an extremity without demonstrable injury to a nerve trunk. Occasionally the trauma may be so slight that the patient does not recollect it. In a few of the cases of reflex sympathetic dystrophy bone atrophy may occur in the region of, or distal to, the site of injury; this local osteoporosis is known as Sudeck's atrophy.

The sufferer complains of persistent pain and tenderness of the affected limb. The pain occurs in hands or feet, and it is diffuse and not confined to the distribution of the damaged nerve trunk. It is usual for the symptom to develop some time after the injury and to increase gradually in intensity. Trigger areas may cause exacerbation of pain, and hyperesthesia and parathesias may be present. The pain prevents use of the hand or foot, which is held motionless and flexed to guard it from any stimulus. The extremity is cold and often slightly swollen; it may be pale or cyanosed. Very often the skin is moist with perspiration (Fig. 9-10). In chronic cases, flexor deformities develop and greater physical impairment results. As this occurs the continuous misery of the chronic pain overwhelms the patient, and the bitterness of failure affects his doctor; the patient is then likely to be labelled psychoneurotic. When relief of the pain does occur the patient's psychoneurosis usually disappears.

Though reflex sympathetic dystrophy is usually classed with vascular disease because of the alleged vasomotor imbalance, the syndrome is essentially one of neural dysfunction with secondary vascular changes. The vasoconstriction, swelling, hyperhydrosis

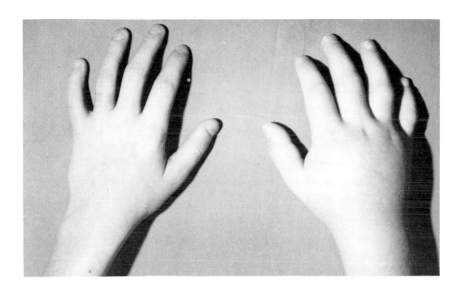

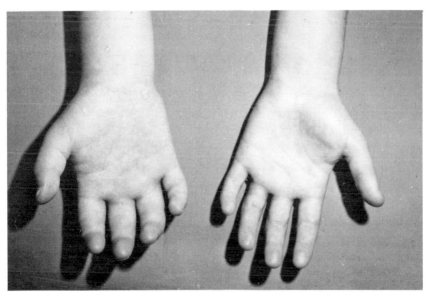

Fig. 9-10. Hands of a girl of 18 with reflex sympathetic dystrophy of the right hand. This was subsequently cured by physiotherapy and sympathectomy.

and osseous changes in the limb are commonly ascribed to autonomic dysfunction and trophic changes, though objective evidence to support these opinions is difficult to obtain. The role of immobility and reflex response to pain may play a large part in their causation. Sympathetic innervation is undoubtedly implicated in the causation of the pain because sympathetic block almost consistently affords relief. Various theories have been put forward to account for the symptom of causalgia. Doupe et al. have suggested that the pain results from an increase in the excitability of sensory nerve endings brought about by sympathetic nerve activity.

The sooner treatment is started the better. The patient should remain in a warm environment and use his painful limb as much as possible. Physiotherapy with warm whirlpool baths, light massage of the muscles, heat and passive and active exercises administered by a firm and sympathetic physiotherapist are of great help. Analgesics should be used sparingly because of the danger of dependance and addiction. Encouragement must be continuous. If these measures are slow in causing improvement, a series of procaine anesthetizations of the regional sympathetic ganglia will often permanently relieve the pain. The therapeutic sympathetic blocks are useful also as a diagnostic measure to test the probable result from sympathectomy which should be carried out if the blocks fail to provide permanent relief.

REFERENCES

Classification of Vascular Diseases

Alarcón-Segovia, D. and Brown, A.L.: Classification and etiological aspects of necrotizing angiitides: An analytic approach to a confused subject with a critical review of the evidence for hypersensitivity of polyarteritis nodosa. Mayo Clinic Proc., *39*:205, 1964.

Scleroderma

Holling, H.E.: Editorial comment on Scharer, L. and Smith, D.W.: Resorption of the terminal phalanges in scleroderma. Arth. and Rheum., *12*:51, 1969.

Norton, W.L. and Nardo, J.M.: Vascular disease in progressive systemic sclerosis (scleroderma). Ann. Int. Med., *73*:317, 1970.
Sackner, M.A.: Scleroderma. Modern Medical Monographs. New York, Grune and Stratton, 1966.

Thromboangiitis Obliterans

McKusick, V.A., et al.: Buerger's disease: a distinct clinical and pathological entity. JAMA, *181*:5, 1962.
Wessler, S., Ming, S.C., Gurewich, V., Freiman, D.G.: A critical evaluation of thrombo-angiitis obliterans. The case against Buerger's disease. New Eng. J. Med., *262*:1149, 1960.

Temporal Arteritis and Polymyalgia Rheumatica

Dixon, A.J.: Polymyalgia Rheumatica. J. Roy. Coll. Physicians London, *4*:55, 1969.

Periarteritis Nodosa

Dornfeld, L., Lecky, J.W., and Peter, J.B.: Polyarteritis and internal renal artery aneurysms. JAMA, *215*:1950, 1971.
Frohnert, P.P., Sheps, S.G.: Long term follow-up study of periarteritis nodosa. Amer. J. Med., *43*:8, 1967.
Kussmaul, A. and Maier, R.: Ueber eine bisher nicht beschrieben eigenthumlickhe Arterienerkrankung (Periarteritis Nodosa), die mit Morbus Brightii und rapid fortschreitender allgemeiner Muskellahmung einhergeht. Deutsches Arch. Klin. Med., *1*:484, 1866.
Rose, G.A. and Spencer, H.: Polyarteritis nodosa. Quart. J. Med., [n.s.] *26*:43, 1957.

Pulseless Disease

McKusick, V.A.: A form of vascular disease relatively frequent in the Orient. Amer. Heart J., *63*:57, 1962.
Roberts, W.C., et al.: The prepulseless phase of pulseless disease, or pulseless disease with pulses. Amer. J. Med., *46*:313, 1969.
Sana, K., Aiba, T., Saito, I.: Angiography in pulseless disease. Radiology, *94*:69, 1970.
Sano, K. and Saito, I.: Immunological studies of pulseless disease. Neurol. Med. Chir., *8*:28, 1966.

Systemic Lupus Erythematosus

Estes, D. and Christian, C.L.: The natural history of systemic lupus erythematosus by prospective analysis. Medicine, *50*:85, 1971.

Hughes, G.R.V.: Significance of anti-DNA antibodies in systemic lupus erythematosus. Lancet, *2*:861, 1971.

Vasculitis

McCombs, R.P.: Systemic "allergic" vasculitis: clinical and pathological relationships. JAMA, *194*:157, 1965.

Scott, J.T., Elsallab, R.A., Laws, J.W.: Digital artery design in rheumatoid arthritis—further observations. Brit. J. Radiol., *40*:748, 1967.

Polycythemia Vera

Chievitz, E. and Thiele, T.: Complications and causes of death in polycythemia vera. Acta. Med. Scandinav., *172*:513, 1962.

Edwards, E.A. and Colley, M.H.: Peripheral vascular symptoms of the initial manifestation of polycythemia vera. JAMA, *214*:1463, 1970.

Vreeken, J., Van Aken, W.G.: Spontaneous aggregation of blood platelets as cause of idiopathic thrombosis and recurrent painful toes and fingers. Lancet, *2*:1394, 1971.

Post-traumatic Reflex Sympathetic Dystrophy

Doupe, J., Cullen, R.H., and Chance, C.O.: Post-traumatic pain and causalgic syndrome. J. Neurol., Neurosurg. and Psychiat., *7*:33, 1944.

Mitchell, S.W., Morehouse, G.R., and Keen, W.W.: Gunshot wounds and other injuries of nerves. Philadelphia, J. B. Lippincott, 1864.

Part IV

DISORDERS OF
VEINS AND LYMPHATICS

10

Disorders of Veins

Most disorders of veins are the result of thrombosis of blood within them, so it is pertinent to ask which factors promote venous thrombosis and which counteract it. Virchow's triad of stasis, hypercoagulability, and intimal change are well recognized as factors which promote thrombosis. Platelet aggregation is a factor which initiates thrombosis, and fibrinolytic activity, one which counteracts it. An increased tendency to venous thrombosis has long been recognized as associated with major surgery, and with this tendency is found an increase in platelet numbers and adhesiveness, an increase in fibrinogen concentration, and a fall in fibrinolytic activity, though these changes occur whether thrombosis occurs or not. Still to be explained are the mechanisms which promote venous thrombosis in estrogen therapy, in homocystinuria, and in females with types A, AB and B, rather than type O blood.

ACUTE VENOUS THROMBOSIS

Prevention

The important precipitating factor of thrombosis is slowing of venous blood flow and stasis of blood in the veins. If venous thrombosis and embolism are to be prevented therefore, patients should not be allowed to remain long in bed. Early mobilization of postoperative and postpartum patients has been a notable development in treatment during the last few years. Much still remains to be done in stimulating medical and nursing staff to encourage bedridden old ladies to change position frequently, even when they have been moved from bed to chair; in fact, prolonged sitting in a chair may be even more dangerous than prolonged lying in a bed because of the greater degree of stasis in the dependent legs. The Lounges and dining tables could be more frequently provided in hospitals to encourage more activity in ambulant patients.

It is not always possible to mobilize patients to the extent which might be desirable. A useful measure to provide some protection during 24 hours is knee-high elastic supports (embolism stockings). They must be well fitting, but an external pressure of 20 mm. Hg at the ankle and 12 mm. Hg at the knee is sufficient. The value of these supports is that they reduce the venous pool in the calf and accelerate venous return both in the bedfast patient and in the ambulant patient.

The disadvantages of routine prophylactic anticoagulation of patients at the risk of thrombosis and embolism must be balanced against the advantages of the procedure. Over the whole range of patients the drawbacks of such action are liable to outweigh the advantages. In certain conditions, such as fracture of the hip in the elderly, it may be that prophylactic anticoagulation is advantageous. For most patients it is better to be alert to the first suspicion of thrombosis. If thrombosis is suspected the patient can be treated with antithrombotic medications, even if the diagnosis of thrombosis remains short of being proven.

Other possible means of preventing postoperative deep venous thrombosis still under investigation are: pharmacological stimulation of endogenous fibrinolysis, and impedance of platelet aggregation by the use of intravenous dextran, or dipyridamole or by small intravenous doses of heparin (1 unit per kg.) repeated half-hourly.

Clinical Diagnosis of Venous Thrombosis

The inexperienced student may be confused by the many signs which are taught him as being valuable in the diagnosis of venous thrombosis. The relative value of these signs is better appreciated if the changes which give rise to them are also considered.

Early Indications. Blood may clot in a vein quietly. When it has done so, the fluid blood is converted to a firm gel which can be felt in a superficial vein. Occasionally a thickened vein wall gives the impression of a blood clot, but usually the sign is unmistakable in a vein which is easily felt. We have no other clinical means of detecting early clot in a deep vein unless it is extensive enough to impede venous return or until its resolution begins. This is unfortunate because it is the freshly formed clot in the deep vein which gives rise to pulmonary emboli rather than the clot which is undergoing resolution. The clinical signs which lead one to suspect the possibility of recent thrombosis are nonspecific. The patient may have an unusual rise of pulse or temperature, or may have nothing more than a recently developed feeling of uneasiness or apprehension. More specifically one leg may be uncomfortable, or there may be an ache in the chest with an increased rate of respiration or some cardiac irregularity. Prompt administration of antithrombotic treatment on such grounds for suspicion may lack the drama of a Trendelenberg operation, but is more likely to be lifesaving.

Venous Obstruction. If clotting is sufficiently extensive to impede the circulation in the leg, venous stasis occurs. This is recognized by peripheral cyanosis, dilated veins, and edema. Cyanosis may be absent or difficult to detect in artificial light. Dilatation of the veins and increased pressure within them is recognized by demonstration that the veins do not collapse when held above heart level. This sign is often useful in the upper limbs, but in the lower limbs edema often obscures the veins and diminishes its value. It is edema, however, which is the most valuable sign of deep venous thrombosis. Even small amounts of edema are not difficult to recognize if the limb is compared with its fellow; the skin looks shinier and more moist, and the appearance of an increase in girth is confirmed by means of a tape measure. Since edema fluid drains downward the degree of swelling is usually greater in the ankle than in the calf; should measurement show the calf to be disproportionally swollen, alternate diagnosis should be considered. Often the affected limb is warmer than its fellow; the cause of this sign is not clear, but it may be the result of slowed passage of blood through the venules. This sign may mislead, and if the increase in skin temperature is very marked, other diagnoses such as cellulitis, are more likely.

Recognition of Phlebitis. Though veins are sensitive to stimuli, they do not appear to respond to clot within them until resolution of the clot begins to occur. Resolution of blood clot is a form of sterile inflammation as is shown by the warmer, redder skin over the resolving thrombus in a superficial vein. In a deep vein resolution is manifested by an ache or pain localized around the veins and increased tone in the surrounding muscles. Light palpation over the superficial veins, and firm palpation over the deep veins elicits tenderness over the course of the veins. Pressure may be applied in a less discriminate manner by means of a blood pressure cuff or muscular contraction (Homan's sign). The first of these methods at the best gives an objective measure of the pressure required to elicit tenderness; the second method (bastard since Dr. Homan is reported to disown it) has little value and is more often misleading than helpful.

Relative Value of Different Signs. The relative value of the above signs in detecting venous thrombosis is hard to assess, since we have no sure way to determine the absence or presence of thrombosis in many cases. In one attempt to determine the value of these tests, all patients admitted to a service were carefully examined for evidence of venous thrombosis and the results were recorded. Some of the patients came to autopsy and special attention was paid to the presence or absence of thrombus in the iliac and femoral and saphenous veins. The results of the antemortem tests were compared with the findings at postmortem and their value assessed by that criterion. Unilateral ankle swelling was found to be the most sensitive test, having detected the majority of cases of thrombosis; it seldom misled. Local tenderness of a vein and increase in skin temperature were also helpful, but to a lesser degree, and were more often misleading. Homan's test and cuff pressure were found to be insensitive and even more frequently misleading.

Instrumental Methods of Detecting Venous Thrombosis

Instrumental methods of diagnosing venous thrombosis have the inherent disadvantage that they are likely not to be available to the house man on his night round, or to the doctor in practice, when a prompt decision of whether or not to anticoagulate the patient is required.

Venography. Venography depends on negative evidence, i.e., that the opaque material does not enter a particular segment of vein. Such failure may occur because of a streamlining effect of the dye past the opening of a vein, or perhaps the section of vein was never developed. Our experience with venography has been limited, but I cannot recall a case of suspected acute venous thrombosis in which the investigation was helpful.

Isotope Tagging. An ingenious method of detecting thrombosis to label fibrinogen (or an antibody to fibrinogen) with a radioisotope. When blood clot forms within a vessel the isotope is concentrated in the fibrin and can be detected by a counter. This method of detecting thrombosis has been valuable in showing the incidence of venous thrombosis after surgery and has further shown the limitation of clinical signs of venous thrombosis. It does not appear to be of general clinical value because it detects thromboses which are not clinically important. It is impractical as a general test because it requires that the iodine uptake of the thyroid gland should be blocked by administration of iodine a day prior to the test. There is also some danger of allergic reactions and transmission of infectious hepatitis.

Ultrasound. One of the more promising methods of detecting obstruction in a vein is by means of the ultrasound. This method depends on the physical fact that reflection of a beam of sound from a stream of flowing blood will be of a different frequency (Doppler Effect), the difference depending on the velocity of the blood stream. In the hands of an expert it gives impressive results, and has the great advantage that it can be carried out at the bedside. But it has not come into wide use, and I suspect that the skill required to interpret the results is somewhat difficult to acquire.

Differential Diagnosis of Acute Venous Thrombosis

In the diagnosis of venous thrombosis it is reasonable to be influenced by the attending circumstances; a postoperative, postpartum, or a patient with cardiac failure and restricted activity is liable to develop venous thrombosis, an active person is much less likely to do so.

A recent study showed that thrombosis of the calf veins occurred in one third of a series of postoperative patients and that it was seldom associated with abnormal symptoms or signs. In this study thrombosis was recognized by means of I_{131}-labelled fibrinogen, and confirmed by phlebography. The implication is that the patient at risk of venous thrombosis, i.e., the postpartum or postoperative patient, is likely to have it, even in the absence of signs, so that if the condition is suspected anticoagulant treatment is likely to be beneficial. However, one should be just as prompt to discontinue the treatment as to start it once the acute condition has subsided.

When thrombosis is suspected in an otherwise healthy person alternate diagnoses should be considered very carefully before starting anticoagulant treatment. Pulmonary embolus is certainly less likely in these patients than in hospitalized patients, so the urgency of treatment is less compelling. I have seen young wives with passing aches in their legs and maybe a fleeting pain in their chests diagnosed as having "phlebitis." When taken off their anovulatory pill and put on anticoagulant therapy, they were subjected not only to the risks of pregnancy and anticoagulant therapy, but the dire threat of a pulmonary embolus was added to their concerns, without alternate diagnoses being given due consideration. The wives of doctors seem to be particularly liable to such poor management.

Phlebodynia. My opinions on the differential diagnosis of acute phlebitis are based on a medical practice in and around a large teaching hospital, so the proportion of nurses and technicians in the practice is rather large. In these circumstances the concept of "phlebodynia" has seemed particularly useful.

This condition is not yet clearly defined, but being alert to the possibility of its occurrence may prevent much iatrogenic disease. A few years ago I became aware of it when a neighboring hospital had an outbreak of "epidemic thrombophlebitis" in the nursing staff. This was so severe that at one time one third of the nurses were off duty. The complaint was of an aching leg. Tenderness was found along the course of a vein which could sometimes be felt as a thickened cord, though the local discoloration which so often marks a superficial thrombophlebitis was absent. There was little or no edema. Occasionally the patient complained of chest discomfort, but not more frequently than might be expected in a group of nurses well aware of the association between thrombosis and pulmonary embolism. In no case was definitive evidence of pulmonary embolus found. Anovulatory pills did not appear to be implicated for a few males had been affected. Heparin therapy had not been beneficial and had caused the usual incidence of unwelcome side effects. Discomfort associated with the disorder was more protracted than would have been the case with a group of cases of venous thrombosis. Similar epidemics had been reported previously. The condition had been considered as an inflammation of the vein wall rather than as intravenous thrombosis. The name phlebodynia had been suggested by comparison with pleurodynia. A viral cause was suggested, but no pathogen had been cultured from the vein walls.

Since becoming aware of this disorder in epidemic form, I have recognized its sporadic occurrence in the general public. The affected often do not consult a physician thinking that the discomfort in their legs is due to a muscular strain or perhaps fearing that if they do consult a physician they will be put onto an unhelpful course of anticoagulant therapy. Two important points in the differentiation of this condition are its insidious onset and the absence of swelling. In the management of such a case, it is important to explain the condition fully and the lack of danger of pulmonary embolus. Analgesics in different strengths may be required, and the patient should be encouraged to remain active.

Other Conditions. A history of trauma, recognition of unusual distribution of swelling, or an undue degree of skin warmth may divert one from a diagnosis of acute venous thrombosis. In three months in a general hospital I saw patients with the following conditions which had originally been misdiagnosed, albeit briefly and tentatively, as acute phlebitis: rupture of the plantaris tendon, shower of emboli from a popliteal aneurysm, prepatellar bursitis and cellulitis, recurrent crysipelas of the leg associated with a chronic fungal infection, acute arthritis of the ankle. In each case the true condition was readily recognized when an alternative diagnosis to acute phlebitis was considered.

Treatment

Management. Bed rest is usually required unless the thrombosis is small and superficial. The rest need not be absolute and the patient is allowed bathroom privileges if he wishes them, for enforcement of strict bed rest in the interest of preventing emboli has the disadvantage of encouraging further thrombosis by promoting stasis.

Elevation of the legs, warm applications, wrapping the limbs with ACE bandages may all give some comfort but need not be insisted on unless they do.

Medication. Of analgesics aspirin has the reputed property of diminishing the agglutination of platelets. Propoxyphene or oxycodone may be required. Sometimes the anti-inflammatory properties of phenylbutazone may be of value.

Anticoagulant Therapy. The main purpose of anticoagulation therapy is to check the extension of thrombosis. There is a choice of heparin or coumadin derivatives. Heparin, in addition to its anticoagulant properties, appears to have some anti-inflammatory action. Coumadin derivatives do not appear to possess this property, for often a patient with acute phlebitis will complain of a return of discomfort in his leg when coumadin is substituted for heparin.

Heparin is best given intravenously to reduce the patient's discomfort and complications. Continuous infusion may be difficult to control, but the use of a heparin lock intravenous needle has proved a useful means of giving injections every 4 to 6 hours. If heparin is given subcutaneously the needle should be fine and sharp and the concentration high. Heparin is available in three strengths: 1,000 units per ml., 5,000 units per ml., and 20,000 units per ml. (100 units is 1 mg.). The standard dose for males is up to 15,000 units, for females, 10,000 units. A course is started with injections at 4 and 8 hours, and continued with doses varying between 5,000 and 12,500 units every 6 hours for 6 days, then every 12 hours for 3 days. It is not strictly necessary to determine clotting times unless there is a suspicion of heparin resistance. If anticoagulation is required for more than 10 days it is usual to switch to coumadin, though occasionally it may be decided to continue a patient on heparin therapy. In addition to the bleeding tendency, a patient on long term heparin is liable to baldness and osteoporosis.

Heparin therapy requires special care. Attendants must be aware that parenteral injections should be avoided but, if necessary must be given with the same care that heparin injections are given. Further, it is preferable to give them about an hour before the next heparin injection is required to avoid the period of peak heparin effect. Old ladies are particularly susceptible to complications of heparin therapy, for in them injections into the buttocks may result in bleeding into the hips and groins or into the retroperitoneal space resulting in femoral nerve entrapment. In a recent study 11 women (average age 61 years) of a group of 42 receiving intravenous heparin therapy had major bleeding episodes, and seven were considered to have had minor bleeding episodes. Of a larger group of men only 4.8 per cent developed major bleeding episodes. Congestive heart failure appeared to be a contributing factor in these complications. In patients on heparin therapy pain and weakness in hip or thigh must be regarded as a first warning of bleeding.

Coumadin derivatives may be used instead of heparin in acute thrombosis. They have been shown to reduce the incidence of thrombosis and pulmonary emboli in a comparative series of older patients with fractured hip and are often used in this manner by orthopedic surgeons. It is doubtful, however, whether they are as effective as heparin in preventing thrombosis. In a series of 11 patients with phlegmasia cerulea dolens seen at the Mayo Clinic, no less than six had been on therapeutic coumadin when the thrombosis progressed.

If long term anticoagulant therapy has been decided on in a case of acute phlebitis, it is usual to change from heparin to coumadin at the end of 10 days. Warfarin sodium (Coumadin) is given in an initial dose of 35 to 60 mg. except when the patient is small, when half that dose is given. Therapeutic depression of prothrombin activity may be expected in 48 hours. The daily maintenance dose is usually between 2.5 and 7.5 mg. but requires checking by means of prothrombin time determinations, which should be maintained in the range of 17 to 30 per cent.

There are no fixed rules to decide how long a patient should be continued on anticoagulant therapy for venous thrombosis. If the thrombosis occurred in association with a transient state of hypercoagulability, a surgical operation or childbirth, there would seem to be no point in continuing anticoagulant therapy over the acute period. If the thrombosis occurred with no obvious cause, a period of 3 months anticoagulation might be of value.

A physician must be aware of the interactions of other drugs on the anticoagulant action of coumadin. Phenylbutazone, oxyphenylbutazone, diphenylhydantoin, and salicylates each potentiate the anticoagulant effect so that the dosage may have to be reduced. On the other hand phenobarbital, chloral, glutethimide, meprobamate, griseofulvin and haloperidol accelerate the inactivation of coumadin so that during their use the dosage of coumadin is steadily increased with the danger that when they are discontinued a severe anticoagulant effect may be experienced.

Experimental Therapy. One means of preventing the extension of thrombosis is to defibrinate the circulating blood. In recent years the effects of defibrination have been recognized in the condition of consumptive coagulopathy and in the effects of the venom of the Malayan pit viper ("pit" refers to a depression in the viper's skull). The active defibrinator in the venom has been extracted as a glycoprotein called ancrod. The substance has low antigenicity and when given intravenously removes about 60 per cent of the fibrinogen from the blood stream. The fibrinogen is converted to an imperfect fibrin polymer which breaks up easily in the circulation and is not deposited in the kidneys as is the fibrin in microangiopathic anemia and consumptive coagulopathy. Early reports indicate that 70 per cent of cases of various thromboses treated with ancrod respond satisfactorily, and in 10 per cent the result were unsatisfactory. Even in the successful cases the treatment must be combined with anticoagulation, and antibodies to ancrod are stimulated over the period of treatment. Recent studies indicate that this therapy has no decided advantage over heparin therapy and is much more expensive.

Treatment with fibrinolysins has the theoretical advantage that accelerated removal of the already formed thrombus should occur. Two fibrinolysins presently available for experimental use are streptokinase and urokinase. Streptokinase, being a bacterial antigen rapidly provokes antibody formation. Urokinase is a plasminogen activator extracted from the urine. It has the advantage of being nonantigenic and digesting fibrin more readily than fibrinogen, but it is very expensive. The value of these products is still being determined, but interest in urokinase is diminishing because the medication is costly, not readily available, and does not appear to have any practical advantage over streptokinase.

Surgical Treatment. The past decade has seen a quick rise, and a slow fall, of interest in surgical removal of the freshly formed thrombus from a vein. The procedure has the appeal of direct action against the diseased state, with the possibility of preventing destruction of venous valves by the resolving thrombus. It may be combined with local heparin therapy; heparin infused distally in the affected vein to discouarge rethrombosis. The procedure would seem an ideal one for severe iliofemoral thrombosis but has not been persistently used because of discouraging long term results.

To prevent extension of the thrombus and passage of emboli to the pulmonary circulation, ligation was previously done on saphenous, femoral, and iliac veins, but experience has shown that the only satisfactory level of ligation is at the inferior vena cava, below the entrance of the renal veins. Various means of narrowing the lumen of the vessel instead of closing it, ("plication") have come into use. It has been our practice to employ inferior cava ligation only when adequate heparinization has failed to prevent a pulmonary embolus. The collateral circulation of the vena cava is very distensible. This accounts for the desirable effect that after caval ligation venous incompetence in the lower

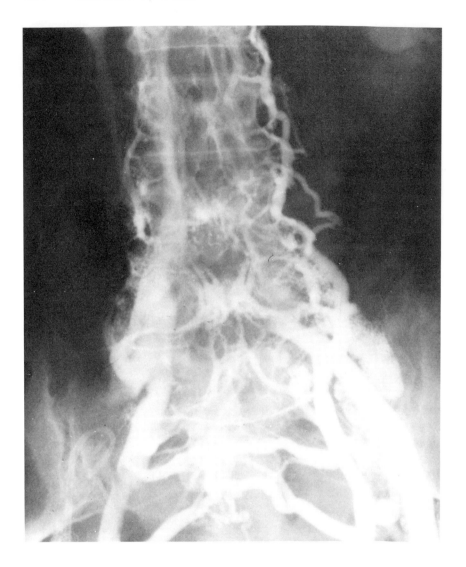

Fig. 10-1. Venogram 18 months after ligation of inferior vena cava showed dilatation of collateral veins.

limbs is less than would be expected (Fig. 10-1) and the undesirable fact that smaller emboli are free to pass from the pelvis and lower extremities to the lungs via this collateral circulation.

Aftermath of Venous Thrombosis

It is instructive to think of two separate processes giving rise to the sequelae of venous thrombosis. One is obstruction of venous return from the limbs, the other is the chronic inflammatory process associated with reorganization of the venous thrombosis. The two processes occur simultaneously in different degrees of severity, but for descriptive purposes it is useful to consider them separately.

Chronic Venous Obstruction and Stasis. When the lower limbs are below heart level the venous return from them is very dependent on muscular movements, even if all the venous valves are competent. In the absence of muscular movements blood accumulates in the feet and calves, the venous pressure rises and edema forms. In health this sequence of events may occur after a long journey in car or airplane, especially under warm conditions.

In sickness such postural edema is seen in patients with rest pain from arterial disease who find they have less discomfort if they sit in a chair rather than lie in bed. It is also seen in patients with neurological or psychiatric diseases which result in prolonged immobility. Frequently these patients are considered to have venous thrombosis, and many do, for the stasis predisposes to thrombosis.

In some, however, the marked changes may be due entirely to stasis. The legs of one such patient are seen in Fig. 10-2. This patient sat in a chair and mourned that she was a widow. Her only movements were to eat and evacuate. Fluid collected in her legs, and she developed stasis dermatitis. When she was first seen it was considered that thrombosis had occurred in her veins. She was not given anticoagulants, but with a regimen of psychotherapy, physiotherapy, and weight reduction the condition of her legs improved remarkably. The absence of leg edema when she resumed normal life indicated that the degree of venous thrombosis had been small.

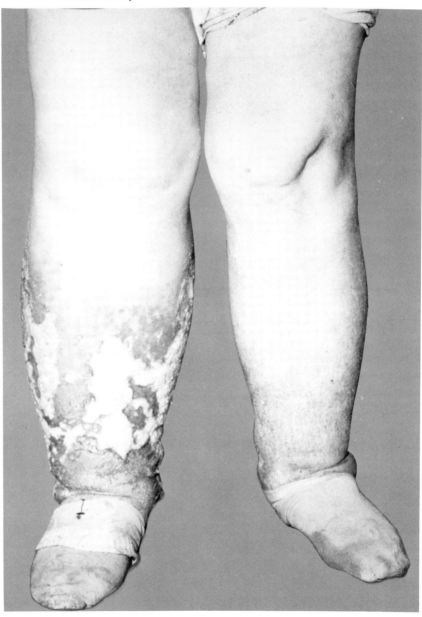

Fig. 10-2a. Stasis dermatitis in an obese, inactive female.

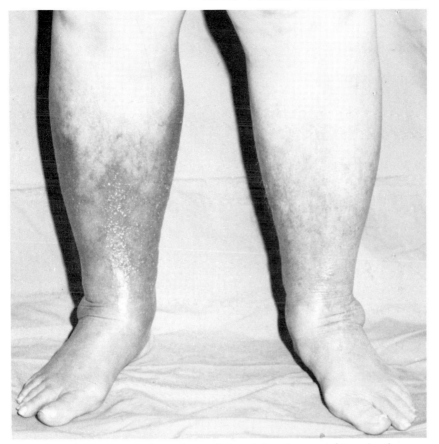

Fig. 10-2b. Resolution of condition following weight reduction and increase in activity.

Following acute venous thrombosis the veins eventually recanalize and collateral pathways dilate. Venous valves involved in the thrombus are likely to be destroyed in the process of resolution and the vein rendered incompetent. The effect of this is seen in swelling and cyanosis of the leg with dilatation of small veins or venules into small caput medusae around the ankle. Venous incompetence is more likely to be troublesome in the patient who does not have the leisure to rest with her feet elevated. Long-standing venous incompetence of the lower extremities leads to breakdown of the skin, first into eczema and then into an ulcer. A venous ulcer is typically just above the medial malleolus. No satisfactory reason has been proposed to explain why the skin should break down just at this point.

By simple treatment much of the distress caused by chronic venous insufficiency can be diminished. No treatment is likely to be effective except that which results in a reduction of the increased venous pressure at the ankle. Bed rest followed by a regimen of adequate daytime rest with legs elevated often results in healing of the ulcer or eczema.

Many therapeutic applications to the eczema and ulcer have been advocated: paraffin gauze, zinc paste, antibiotics and steroids. All should be used with caution because of the danger that their application will render an already damaged skin hypersensitive to them. The result would be an iatrogenic dermatitis. When reading or hearing of the wonderful results of application of this or that salve it is well to remember that reduction of venous pressure is what heals stasis dermatitis and ulcer, not a lotion or an ointment. Elastic stockings are required for comfort and to improve the venous return. Diuretics may be used to reduce the fluid collection,

If the above measures are inadequate to control the cutaneous effects of prolonged stasis, the application of an Unna paste boot or its modern equivalent may be helpful. A bandage in which plastic material is incorporated is wrapped around the leg as a resilient cast and is left in position for a week, after which it is reapplied if necessary.

Occasionally ligation and stripping of the veins may be of use. Whether or not surgery will be likely to help is best decided by determining whether or not the superficial veins are being fed from the deep veins by means of incompetent communicating veins. The tourniquet is used for this decision. The position of the veins is marked by a ballpoint pen and they are then emptied by elevation of the legs. The patient stands and the filling time of the veins is noted. The procedure is then repeated but with the tourniquet lightly applied over the vein to be tested to prevent reflux flow down the superficial veins. If the filling time is appreciably prolonged, it indicates that the superficial vein is not being filled from the deep veins and that its obliteration may help the patient. If full scale ligation and stripping is decided on, the position of incompetent communicating veins should be marked. After years of disfavor the injection treatment with sclerosing substances is being used to a small degree in conjunction with ligation and stripping.

When the ulcer is slow to heal skin grafting may be very helpful once the ulcer base is clean; ideally this should be an autograft, but homografts from a skin bank have been found to be helpful. When bed rest is not feasible the leg should be firmly supported by an elastic bandage or stocking; in the case of the former, the patient, or his attendant must be instructed in the proper technique of bandaging so that the upper part of the bandage is less tight than the lower. Ligation and stripping of the affected veins is likely to be helpful if the tests for competence of the communicating veins so indicate.

Postphlebitis Syndrome. Following an attack of acute venous thrombosis many patients develop a major complaint of aching, tiredness, or burning pain in the affected leg. The severity of the symptoms is not comparable to the objective assessment of venous insufficiency, and indeed may be quite severe though there is no evidence of venous obstruction. Such patients are in danger of being considered as tiresome neurotics. The cause of the persistence of complaints is unknown; they may be due to the sterile inflammation of clot resolution, though it is possible that some low grade infection of the affected veins occurs. This condition of "postphlebitis syndrome" is very like that of "phlebodynia" described in the foregoing section.

The condition is likely to last for 1 to 2 years. Coumadin therapy appears to be without effect on the discomfort, though the patients are often unwilling to stop the drug because of a fear of a pulmonary embolus if they do. This fear appears to have been stimulated unnecessarily. Analgesics suitable for a chronic state are required. Some patients have experienced benefit from a week's course of an antiinflammatory agent phenylbutazone or indomethacin. Some years ago patients appeared to derive benefit from injections of hexamethonium, a ganglion blocker. This drug has now gone out of use but its former use suggests that a trial of sympathetic blockade would be of interest. Currently the most favored method (see section on Raynaud's disease) would be an intra-arterial injection of reserpine.

PHLEGMASIA CERULEA DOLENS AND PHLEGMASIA ALBA DOLENS

These euphonious names are descriptive of two varieties of venous thrombosis. Phlegmasia alba dolens describes acute venous thrombosis with marked edema. When it occurs postpartum it is described as milk leg, perhaps because the condition occurs in a lactating woman or perhaps because of the fanciful notion that milk had drained from breast to leg.

Phlegmasia cerulea dolens should be used only to describe a condition in which intense cyanosis of the affected limb is associated with gangrene of terminal portions. Figure 10-3 shows a typical case. This was the leg of a patient with widespread

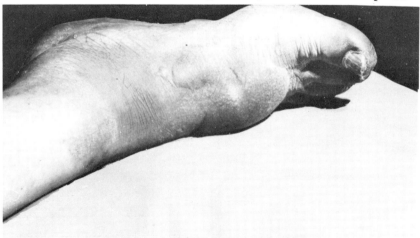

Fig. 10-3. Phlegmasia cerulea dolens in a patient with carcinomatosis secondary to cancer of the breast.

carcinomatosis secondary to cancer of the breast. Differential diagnosis from arterial gangrene was not difficult, for the condition developed slowly. The cyanosed skin proximal to the gangrene was warm, and the dorsalis pedis pulse was beating strongly. The associated pathology appears to be an extension of thrombosis from the veins into the microcirculation. This condition usually, but not invariably, occurs in patients seriously ill from another cause so that the prognosis is poor. However, when it occurs in association with a nonlethal condition, treatment is occasionally successful in maintaining life with a useful limb.

The seriousness of the condition stimulates an all-out treatment effort. First, consideration should be given to the precipitating cause. When phlegmasia cerulea dolens occurs in a patient with a transient precipitating cause, usually surgery or childbirth, the sequence of therapeutic measures should be quickly decided. If the patient is suitable for thrombectomy this should be carried out as soon as possible. Transudation of fluid into the limb may have contributed to a shocklike state; so intravenous replacement of fluid may be required.

An early decision, too, should be made whether a sympathetic block (epidural or paravertebral) will be carried out. This procedure serves the dual purpose of relieving pain and abolishing autonomic vasoconstriction. Following these decisions the patient should be made warm in bed with the leg elevated. Heparin therapy may now be started, and the concern and alarm of the patient dealt with by comforting reassurance, analgesics and tranquilizers. If phlegmasia cerulea dolens occurs in a patient rapidly becoming moribund from a malignant lesion, palliative treatment should be energetically pursued. The most helpful procedure is likely to be an epidural block with plentiful use of tranquilizers. Heparin therapy should be started only if there is a specific indication of pulmonary embolus.

Published figures on the effects of treatment of phlegmasia cerulea dolens may be difficult to assess. If the results appear to be favorable, consider the criteria by which the diagnosis was made, for some authors use this label to cover all patients with venous thrombosis; if the results appear to be unfavorable consider the associated disease condition, which is often of a lethal nature. Whatever the statistics of prognosis, once the decision has been made to treat the condition actively, the physician should appear sanguine in order to transmit his hopefulness to the patient.

VENOUS THROMBOSIS IN THE UPPER LIMB

Conditions which favor venous thrombosis in the lower limb seldom give rise to thrombosis in the upper limbs. Acute venous thrombosis does occur in the upper limb but under circumstances which indicate a different etiology. The patient is more likely to be male than female, young rather than old, and to have carried out undue exertion rather than to have been inactive. The thrombosis is usually in the subclavian vein and is probably due to traumatic compression of the vein at the thoracic outlet, between the clavicle and the first rib. The limb is cyanosed and swells and the increased venous pressure is fairly easily diagnosed.

In a young man with a history of unusual exertion the diagnosis is usually straightforward and the course of the condition satisfactory even with conservative therapy. Pulmonary embolus is very unusual. Beneficial results have been reported to follow thrombectomy and resection of a portion of the first rib by the axillary route. In an older person the more sinister causes of venous obstruction have to be considered. The differential diagnosis of some of these cases provides pitfalls for the unwary. For example, one female, 70 years of age, complained of a recent onset of swelling of the left arm. The venous pressure in the arm and neck was increased. (Fig. 6-2). Axillary or thoracic outlet malignancy was thought to be a likely cause. The venogram showed an apparent obstruction of the subclavian vein with dilatation of the collateral circulation. At this stage a neurologist abashed the experts on vascular disease by demonstrating the presence of the murmur of an A-V fistula. This led to a rapid revision of the clinical and radiological diagnosis. The etiology of the fistula was never determined but was thought to be arteriosclerotic. Another unusual cause of increased brachial venous pressure is idiopathic mediastinal fibrosis.

VARICOSE VEINS

Varicose veins are usually considered as primary and secondary. Primary varicose veins affect the superficial system of the legs of men. The most generally accepted concept is that they develop because of hereditary weakness of the greater saphenous system and its valves, but the orthostatic increase of saphenous vein pressure is another factor, since varicosities are more common in tall men and do not occur in the brachial veins. Cases are seldom referred to physicians since they are judged to be essentially a surgical disorder. Since the deep veins are not involved there is little tendency to edema formation and the dilated veins are well contained by elastic support. If they become symptomatic the patients are best referred for ligation and stripping for the results are good and the danger that dilatation and stasis may progress through the communicating veins to the deep veins resulting in incompetence of both systems is avoided.

Secondary varicose veins are superficial veins which dilate following thrombosis of the deep veins for which they form a collateral channel. Since the deep veins are obstructed, edema forms readily.

ORAL CONTRACEPTIVES

It is generally accepted that the use of oral contraceptive agents is associated with an increase in thromboembolic phenomena. It appears that the estrogen component of the pill is the more active in promoting thrombosis. The risk, however, is a small one compared to other risks at this stage of civilization. From published figures of annual mortality rates for British women of childbearing age Table 10-1 is derived.

Since oral contraceptives offer the most acceptable and effec-

TABLE 10-1. ESTIMATED ANNUAL MORTALITY IN WOMEN
AGES 20 TO 44 YEARS

All causes	97 per 100,000
Maternity	12 per 100,000
Automobile accidents	6 per 100,000
Oral contraceptives	3 per 100,000

tive means of preventing unwanted pregnancy, it follows from the above comparison of mortality that nine maternal lives are saved each year by the use of oral contraceptives, and the efficiency of an alternative method would have to be very high to diminish this lifesaving measure.

Morbidity associated with oral contraceptives is estimated at 47 per 100,000 users, but this figure may well have been inflated by inclusion of sufferers from "phlebodynia" in the figures for thrombophlebitis.

The above findings indicate that the risk from thrombosis in women on estrogen therapy is small and generally acceptable. There are, however, circumstances in which the risk becomes unacceptable. Patients with congenital heart disease and a veno-arterial shunt, and patients with a prosthetic valve in the right ventricle have been found to be extremely prone to accelerated development of obliterative pulmonary artery disease when they are on the pill. The mechanism is presumed to be deposition of platelet thrombi in the small pulmonary vessels. Oral contraceptives are certainly contraindicated in such patients.

So far there have been no reports of an increased incidence of postoperative thrombosis in patients undergoing emergency surgery whilst on contraceptives, nor does it appear to be the practice to cease taking the pill when being prepared for an elective operation.

MALIGNANCY AND THROMBOPHLEBITIS

A hundred years ago Trousseau reported on the increased incidence of thrombophlebitis in carcinoma of the pancreas. Since then migratory phlebitis has been observed to occur in one fifth to one third of patients with carcinoma of the pancreas. The incidence is smaller when the cancer is in the head of the pancreas, and greater when it is in the tail; in other words, there is a higher incidence with malignant mucinous carcinoma, and a lower incidence in association with obstructive jaundice. The thromboses are superficial and migratory, and are not prevented by anticoagulant therapy. These observations represent the basis of the so-called Trousseau's sign of malignancy. The sign is of doubtful clinical value and it is doubtful that it has ever led to the diagnosis of an operable cancer.

REFERENCES

Detection of Postsurgical Thrombosis

Sigal, B., et al.: Doppler ultrasound for occlusion of deep veins due to thrombosis and incompetent valves associated with post-phlebitic syndrome. Arch. Surg., *100*:535, 1970.

Wheeler, H.B., Mullick, S.C., Anderson, J.N. and Pearson, D.: Diagnosis of occult deep vein thrombosis by a non-invasive bedside technique. Surgery, *70*:20, 1971.

Prevention of Postsurgical Thrombosis

Kakkar, V.V., et al.: Low doses of heparin in prevention of deep vein thrombosis. Lancet, *2*:671, 1971.

Phlebodynia

Brosius, G.R., Calvert, M.D., and Chin, T.D.Y.: Epidemic phlebodynia. Arch. Int. Med., *108*:442, 1961.

Browse, N.L.: The painful deep-vein syndrome. Lancet, *1*:1251, 1970.

Pearson, J.S.: Phlebodynia. Circulation, *7*:370, 1953.

Embolism Stockings

Husni, E.A., Ximenes, J.O.C., Goyette E.D.: Elastic support of lower limbs in hospital patients. A critical study. JAMA, *214*:1456, 1970.

Wilkins, R.W., Mixler, G., Stanton, J.R. and Litter J.: Elastic stockings in the prevention of pulmonary embolism. A preliminary report. New Eng. J. Med., *246*:360, 1956.

Complications of Heparin Therapy

Vieweg, W.V.R., Piscatelli, R.L., Houser, J.J.H. and Proulx, R.A.: Complications of intravenous administration of heparin in elderly women. JAMA, *213*:1303, 1970.

11

Lymphatic Disorders of the Limbs

TABLE 11-1. CLASSIFICATION OF LYMPHATIC DISORDERS

INFLAMMATORY (lymphangiitis)
> Streptococcal
> Postphlebitic syndrome
> Trichophytosis

OBSTRUCTIVE (lymphedema)

> *Primary:*
>> Congenital (Milroy)
>> Hereditary (Meige)
>> Lymphedema precox
>> Spontaneous lymphedema

> *Secondary:*
>> Chronic inflammatory: recurrent lymphangiitis, filariasis
>> Sclerosing retroperitonitis or mediastinitis
>> Malignant invasion
>> Surgical excision of lymph nodes
>> Radiation therapy

TUMORS OF LYMPH VESSELS
> Simple or capillary
> Cavernous
> Cystic (cystic hygroma)

INFLAMMATORY

Lymphatics drain inflammatory agents and products from the tissue spaces into the lymph nodes where bacteriocidal and immunological processes render the agents and their products innocuous. Subclinical lymphangiitis may therefore be considered as a continuing protective process of the body.

Acute Ascending Lymphangiitis

Ascending lymphangiitis results from a puncture wound of the skin which permits invasion of the tissues by organisms which are

227

usually β-hemolytic streptococci. The organisms pass into the lymphatics and on into the bloodstream. Pathologists and their assistants who perform autopsies, and commercial meat handlers are particularly susceptible to this danger. Before the introduction of sulfonamides and antibiotics, this infection was often fatal and greatly feared. Adequate therapy has greatly diminished the seriousness of the condition.

The wound is small with little local reaction, but the general bodily reaction of chills and fever is marked. Lymphatics draining the infected area show their course by the presence of a red streak up the limb. The regional lymph nodes are tender and moderately enlarged. Procaine penicillin G, 300,000 to 600,000 units intramuscularly twice a day for 10 days, is the drug of choice for the condition.

Recurrent Lymphangiitis

Some patients are prone to recurrent streptococcal infections of the skin with associated lymphangiitis. The infection is manifested by circumscribed indurated inflammation of the skin often in the same area and is known as erysipelas.

The recurrent condition is often associated with chronic lymphatic obstruction, sometimes with the postphlebitic syndrome. In both conditions trichophytosis between the toes is often associated. When the condition is associated with chronic venous insufficiency, it may be mistaken for recurrent thrombophlebitis.

Characteristically the recurrence begins with chills and a febrile reaction to 103° to 105° F. (39.4 to 40.6° C.). There is associated headache, nausea, and maybe vomiting. The site of infection is often manifested by a circumscribed area of indurated skin. Red streaks appear up the course of the lymphatics and the local lymph nodes are enlarged and tender. The acute attack is treated as an acute ascending lymphangiitis, but when a patient has experienced several attacks a prophylactic program should be considered as outlined below. If such a program is established subsequent attacks may be averted, or at least greatly reduced in frequency and severity.

TREATMENT OF RECURRENT LYMPHANGIITIS

Hygiene
1. Daily cleansing of feet and hands with pHisohex soap.
2. Treatment of dermophytosis:
   a. Soaks of the feet in potassium permanganate solution 1: 8,000.
   b. Dusting of the feet and hands with Desenex or Mycil powder or use of Desenex ointment.

Control of Lymphedema
1. Elevation of legs whenever possible
2. Elastic stockings
3. Intermittent use of diuretics: thiazide, furosemide, ethacrynic acid
4. Use of a device which rhythmically compresses the limb

Control of Infections
1. Oral: potassium phenoxymethyl penicillin, 125 to 250 mg., or if the patient is allergic to penicillin, Erythromycin 250 mg. These doses are to be given 4 times daily for 1 week in 4.
2. Parenteral benzathine penicillin G (Bicillin), 1,200,000 units intramuscularly once a month.

OBSTRUCTIVE LYMPHEDEMA

Primary Lymphedema

Primary or idiopathic lymphedema (lymphedema praecox) is due to stasis of tissue fluid in the tissues of the limbs resulting in persistent swelling of the part. It is more frequently encountered in women than in men. The term praecox refers to early development, for in the majority of cases the condition appears with the adolescent spurt of growth at puberty, though it may appear as early as 9 years or be delayed as late as 25, or even middle life. One lower extremity is usually affected, both are more seldom affected, and an upper extremity rarely. There is no evidence that the condition shortens the expected life span.

The patient is usually in her late teens or early twenties when she becomes aware of a tendency of one ankle to swell by the end of the day. At first the swelling has disappeared by the morning but becomes noticeable again during the day. The swelling is more apparent in hot weather and, in some female patients is worse during the days which immediately precede the menstrual flow. The condition progresses slowly and the extent and degree of swelling increases over a period of months or years. In some cases the edema may progress more rapidly so that the whole leg becomes involved within a month or so. In others the swelling may remain limited to the calf and does not extend above the knee. In fortunate cases the swelling may progress for a while and then after a year or so reach a steady state. Spontaneous regression is rare but has been reported in cases where the condition is associated with Turner's syndrome.

In the early stages the edema will pit with finger pressure and largely subside with bed rest, but with the passage of time when lymph stasis has provoked a fibroblastic reaction in the subcutaneous tissues the edema becomes resistant to finger pressure and subsides little with bed rest. The overlying skin becomes roughened and sometimes verruciform (Fig. 11-1). In severe cases small blebs of lymph appear on the skin surface which discharge their contents and are likely to become infected. In the later stages infection of the skin with recurrent cellulitis is common. Ulceration of the skin occurs with the areas of inflammation, but ulcers of the type seen in venous incompetence do not occur.

Even when the limb has increased in size to elephantine proportions the absence of discomfort and pain is in contrast to the continuous discomfort and complaints of a patient with chronic thrombophlebitis or postphlebitic syndrome. A dull heavy sensation may be present which may result from the ponderous limb. It is the unesthetic appearance of the thick ankles which first brings the patient to the doctor for the whole limb is liable to become edematous with obliteration of the normal contours. Thick ankles distress the female patient particularly and the male patient resents that he cannot wear the fashionably tight pants.

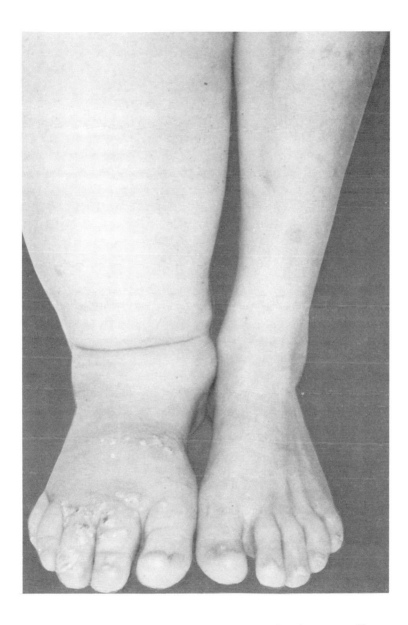

Fig. 11-1. Lymphedema praecox of left leg showing verruciform eruption of the foot from which lymph oozed.

The foot is less involved so that a different size of footwear for each foot is seldom required.

Congenital and Hereditary Lymphedema

Congenital lymphedema, as its name implies, is present at birth as edema of a foot, leg, or thigh, though it may not be noticed by the parents until the child is several months old. Milroy (1892) is usually given eponymic precedence for this disorder though Nonne (1891) had preceded him with a description of a family in which edema was present at birth. The cause of this early appearance of lymphedema is not known, though in some cases annular zones of sclerosis are present above the edematous area of the limb. It has been suggested that these zones are the result of pressure of amniotic bands during fetal life.

In 1865, Letessier had described a familial form of lymphedema in which the onset of lymphedema was delayed until later in life, most often at puberty. Meige described a similar family in 1898, and usually this form of hereditary lymphedema is known as Meige's disease. It is not clear whether these are two discrete forms of lymphedema. They differ neither in pathology nor in the form of inheritance, and both are very rarely seen in practice. Omitting the history of inheritance, when the affected child reaches puberty, the clinical features of the condition are the same as those of primary lymphedema.

Esterly's account of the genetics of hereditary lymphedema is the most recent and thorough. He proposes that the disorder is inherited as a dominant trait, most frequently as a simple autosomal dominant with complete penetrance but variable expressivity. Since congenital hereditary lymphedema occasionally occurs in lower animals, it has been possible to carry out controlled observations on its transmission in them. In cattle and swine the disorder is reported to be inherited as an autosomal recessive trait, but in the dog Patterson found the transmission to be, as in the human, a dominant trait. The expressivity is found to be as variable as in man, and the occurrence of apparent skipped generations may be due to mildly affected persons who escape clinical detection.

In the human families reported the overall male to female ratio is 66:81, but within transmitted sibships the ratio rises to 33:47. This female predominance suggests some form of sex inheritance but evidence of specific male to male transmission and unaffected daughters of affected males excludes X-linked dominant inheritance. Of interest was a study of chromosomes in a series of congenital lymphedema (Benson et al.). Of 32 phenotypic females, 26 had normal karyotypes, 2 had an XO sex chromosome complement, 1 had a ring chromosome replacing one of the "G" group chromosomes in 4 per cent of leukocytes. The authors of this study suggest that chromosome abnormalities should be suspected in congenital lymphedema, especially when there are associated somatic abnormalities such as webbing of the neck. They point out that primary lymphedema may regress spontaneously when associated with Turner's syndrome but otherwise, almost never.

Pathophysiology. In established lymphedema it is not unusual for the volume of the affected limb to be doubled. The true skin and the tissues underlying the deep fascia appear to be normal so that the major increase in this bulk is in the subcutaneous tissues. Comparisons of the volumes of different tissues in the normal limb and the lymphedematous limb show that the volume of the subcutaneous tissues is increased 10 to 20 times.

The protein content of the retained fluid is proportional to the severity of the edema, rising from a normal 0.7 g.% to as much as 3.0 g.%. Dispersal of protein injected into the affected tissues is slowed; I_{131}-tagged albumin injected into the subcutaneous tissues is found to disappear at a rate 10 times slower than in normal skin. Retention of proteins and their breakdown products in the tissue spaces is associated with a fibroblastic invasion which leads to an overgrowth of connective tissues. The subcutaneous fat cells are slowly replaced by fibrous tissue which leads to the brawny nonpitting edema that is characteristic of lymphedema. Atrophy of the overlying skin may occur, but true ulceration is much less common than in venous insufficiency.

Kinmonth has shown that the lymphatics of limbs with primary lymphedema differ from those of the normal limb or of those with secondary lymphedema. By the use of lymphangiography he showed that the abnormal vessels were either hypoplastic, aplastic, or varicose and incompetent. Rather more than one half of the cases of lymphedema show hypoplasia, and in one tenth the hypoplasia is sufficiently severe to be termed aplasia. In one quarter of the cases dilatation of the lymphatic trunks results in a condition of varicosity of the lymphatics. Flow in existing lymphatics might be bidirectional, running, as in the normal, from the superficial dermis to the deeper dermis, but also in the reverse direction—"dermal back flow." In the opinion of Kinmonth this is due to lymph stasis developing in otherwise normal tissues because there is an area of lymphatic stasis or obstruction proximally. An increase in blood flow is often associated with the thickening of the subcutaneous tissues so that the lymphedematous leg often feels hot and inflamed.

DIFFERENTIAL DIAGNOSIS

Venous Obstruction

A simple cause of swelling of the legs of a plump young girl is the wearing of a tight "panty girdle." The edema is mild and more likely to be due to venous obstruction than to lymphatic obstruction though the limbs may not be cyanosed nor the veins prominent. The patient needs to be warned against wearing constricting garments on the body or legs.

Chronic venous insufficiency and lymphedema may be difficult to distinguish when the condition is not severe. Each disorder is likely to affect only one leg. In the early stages of lymphedema the edema pits on pressure and disappears on elevation of the leg as does the edema of venous obstruction. The two disorders may be distinguished by history: the onset of lymphedema is insidious whereas that of venous insufficiency is likely to have appeared in the course of an illness or following childbirth, surgical operation, or the use of oral contraceptives. The two disorders are distinguishable also in that a leg swollen because of lymphedema is remarkably free of discomfort and this contrasts with the discomfort of a leg which is swollen because of venous insufficiency. In venous insufficiency the superficial veins are liable to be distended and often tender and the skin somewhat cyanosed; this contrasts with the smooth pale swelling of lymphedema.

In the advanced stages of venous insufficiency and lymphedema the conditions are even more distinguishable for the thickened skin and firm consistency of established lymphedema contrasts with the soft edema, stasis dermatitis, ulceration, and superficial varicosities of chronic venous insufficiency. It is true that some degree of lymphedema may be superimposed on the condition of chronic venous insufficiency when attacks of recurrent lymphangitis or cellulitis have occurred. Also there are occasional cases in which lymphedema and venous insufficiency coexist. Venograms and lymphangiograms may be used to assess the contribution of each disorder, but such investigations are seldom required.

Secondary Edema

Since edema from most causes affects both legs and many cases of lymphedema affect only one leg, the distinction between lymphedema and edema from other causes is not difficult. Physical examination, blood count, and routine urine test in most cases will suffice to exclude the possibility of renal, hepatic, or cardiac causes of edema. If required, serum electrophoresis will exclude hypoalbuminemia or hyperglobulinemia.

Idiopathic Edema

The syndrome of idiopathic edema is one of which physicians are becoming increasingly aware. It is not an uncommon disorder in females at an age when they are liable to develop lymphedema. It is important to recognize it, not only for differential diagnosis, but also because the two conditions may occur simultaneously and each exacerbate the effects of the other.

The ultimate cause of edema in idiopathic edema is unsure but it is practical to regard it as an abnormal pattern of excretion of sodium and water by the kidneys such that when the patient is upright antidiuresis occurs and diuresis when the patient lies down. This is a reversal of the normal pattern. The roles of excess filtration from the capillaries and secondary aldosteronism remain uncertain. The result of these changes is that fluid is retained over the whole of the body in the daytime, though by the effects of gravity much of the fluid may drain into the legs and so resemble lymphedema.

The patient with idiopathic edema complains of discomfort in the abdomen and legs during the daytime and is aware of swelling of her hands and puffiness of her face. Symptoms tend to regress during nighttime recumbency because the excess fluid is eliminated in a nocturnal diuresis. The severity of the condition tends to be periodic and is often related to the menstrual cycle.

Once the condition is suspected the simplest way of furthering the diagnosis is to have the patient weight herself each day on arising and retiring. Because of the retention of fluid the patient with idiopathic edema with have an unduly large weight gain during the day with an equally large weight loss during the night. A normal person may be expected to gain 0.5 to 1.4 kg. (1 to 3 lb.) during the day so that a weight gain of more than 1.4 kg. (3 lbs.) during a day is strongly suggestive of idiopathic edema. Many times patients will lose several pounds overnight. The cause of the loss and gain of weight becomes apparent when the patient measures her urine output and compares the volume passed between 7 a.m. and 7 p.m. with that passed between 7 p.m. and 7 a.m. Normally the daytime volume exceeds that of the nighttime, but in patients with idiopathic edema there is a nocturnal diuresis and this ratio is reversed. This simple procedure of charting weights and urine volume is diagnostic. It is also an important procedure to instruct the patient in the factors which aggravate her fluid retention and those which relieve it.

The antidiuretic effect may be demonstrated by a simple morning water excretion test done first with the patient lying down and then with the patient up and about. In the first test under fasting conditions the patient drinks 1,500 ml. of water over one half hour. After emptying her bladder she lies down and remains so for four hours except at hourly intervals when she empties her bladder. She must be specifically warned against smoking because of its antidiuretic effect. Normal subjects excrete 300 ml. or more urine in an hour and at least 80 per cent of the ingested water over the four hours. In idiopathic edema this last test should give normal results. In the second test on a subsequent day the patient repeats the test but remains up and about during the ensuing four hours. Patients with idiopathic edema will show a marked decrease in hourly urine output and a decided reduction in the fraction of ingested water which is excreted.

These tests provide the diagnosis but they also indicate an important fact in treatment of the condition, which is that a period of recumbency during the day will enable the patient to excrete some of the retained fluid. Elastic support of the legs which is of value in both idiopathic edema and lymphedema will not, however, in the former condition prevent retention of fluid in the body. General advice to the patient is that she should restrict caloric intake if she is overweight because obesity itself tends to cause retention of fluid. Sodium intake can be restricted to 3 to 5 grams of sodium daily and the diet arranged so that it contains foods high in potassium but low in sodium, such as bananas. There is no need to restrict fluid intake.

Diuretics are of some value. In idiopathic edema spironolactone is useful for it acts as a mild diuretic and also diminishes the secondary hyperaldosteronism which may be present. Spironolactone further facilitates the retention of potassium and enhances the effectiveness of other diuretics. It is given in a daily dose of between 25 and 100 mg. most of which is given in the morning when the patient is likely to be up and about. Additional diuretics such as a thiazide, triamterene, furosemide or ethacrynic acid may be required. Supplementary diuretics are given once every 3 to 5 days at the start of treatment, and the intervals between administration are gradually increased. The patient should be encouraged to lengthen the intervals between taking these diuretics so that the response to them is greater. It is wise to advise drastic reduction of sodium intake in the 24 hours following a diuresis to limit the rebound retention of sodium; to this end a day's existence on rice (unsalted) and fruit is advised.

Potassium supplements are seldom required if diuretic therapy is adequately controlled.

We have found that patients with idiopathic edema tend to be more emotionally upset and obsessive than those with lymphedema alone. They are liable to overdose themselves with diuretics with resultant fatigue, muscular weakness and postural hypotension. They must be warned against this and the effect of therapy on serum potassium and uric acid should be checked.

Treatment can be monitored on the basis of the daily weight recorded in the morning and evening. Encouragement can be given by telling the patient that though lymphedema is likely to persist, the exacerbating cyclic edema is a condition which in most cases runs its course.

Malignant Edema

Fortunately malignant edema is very rare in the young. Swelling of the leg and palpable nodes in the groin suggest malignancy, for the lymph nodes are not characteristically enlarged in lymphedema. Melanoma is the most likely malignancy to arise but undue firmness in the tissues of the leg may indicate sarcoma of the muscle or bone. In the older patient who develops swelling of a limb, malignancy must certainly be considered, if only to be ruled out. The upper extremities are more often involved by this cause of lymphedema in contrast to the lower extremities which are more often the seat of simple lymphedema. Recent development of edema of an upper limb merits serious attention to the possibility of carcinoma of the breast or mediastinal neoplasm or idiopathic mediastinal fibrosis. Swelling of the lower limbs necessitates a thorough pelvic examination and consideration of a retroperitoneal tumor or idiopathic retroperitoneal fibrosis.

Filariasis

Lymphatic obstruction due to infestation by one or more of a numerous species of threadlike nematodes (filariasis) is a chronic condition. The female adult worm living in the tissues of the host gives birth to embryos, known as microfilariae because of their delicate elongated shape (150 to 350μ). The microfilariae migrate in the peripheral bloodstream from where they are taken up by a blood sucking culicine mosquito and transmitted to another human. From the time of infection to the time when the adult female worm produces microfilariae is approximately 1 year, though inflammatory reactions to infection may occur at any time between 1 month and 2 years after exposure to infection. Worms, alive or dead and degenerating, lodge in the lymphatics where they give rise to an inflammatory granulomatous reaction which blocks the lymphatic channel. The infection may run its course over many years and varies greatly in its clinical manifestations. Transfer to cool climate usually diminishes its effects.

In the cases which may be mistaken for idiopathic lymphedema the stay of the individual in the infested area may have been short and the inflammatory symptoms mild. It is therefore worthwhile to inquire into the possibility of having been exposed to infection in all cases of lymphedema, though without repeated infections and notable inflammatory episodes the likelihood of finding filarial infestation is small. Diagnosis, even in the rare case, however, is worthwhile, for the disease can be treated successfully.

Observation of the blood smears for microfilariae is the oldest and best diagnostic test, and specimens are best obtained in the early hours of the evening when the organisms are most numerous in the bloodstream. Sasa recommends taking 30 cmm. of blood in a measured pipette to be spread in three even lines on a glass slide and stained with azure II and eosin. The microfilariae, if present, are recognized under the low power objective. Of serological tests, a soluble antigen fluorescent antibody (SAFA) appears to be the most promising. An antigen has been prepared from the *Dirofilaria immitis* (known as FST antigen) which when injected into the skin gives an immediate wheal and flare type of reaction. This skin test gives an 80 per cent reactor rate in known positives, with a low incidence of false positives. If filariasis is shown to be present, diethyl carbamazine (Hetrazan*) is given to kill off the microfilariae and either kill or permanently sterilize the adult females. 2 mg. per kg. of body weight is given 3 times a

* Trademark, Lederle

day for 1 or 2 weeks. Headache, dizziness, and malaise may be expected during therapy.

LYMPHEDEMA: TREATMENT

The control of lymphedema must be started at an early stage to be effective. The patient and her parents should be reassured that no serious heart or kidney disease is responsible for the edema of the leg. The rationale of treatment must be understood by them; this is that the disorder cannot be cured but that adequate control by means of elastic stockings and diuretics should prevent the condition from getting worse. Failure to do this is liable to result in a progression of the condition with increasing deformity and discomfort. The longer lymphedema remains uncontrolled the more swelling occurs, the more firm the fibrosis, and the less the condition can be controlled.

Diuretics are of considerable value in the control of lymphedema. Hydrochlorothiazide, 50 mg. taken daily, will help to maintain elimination of excess fluid though in more resistant cases furosemide or ethacrynic acid may be more effective. The patient needs to be instructed in the proper use of diuretics and avoidance of electrolyte disturbance and under-hydration resulting from their abuse. Symptoms of overdosage are lethargy, muscular weakness and cramps. For the first few months on diuretic therapy their effect may be monitored by occasional determination of serum electrolytes and thereafter by checking the patient's weight.

To contain the edema, elastic support of the legs is in effect comparable to its use in venous insufficiency. Compression of the leg results in an increase of tissue pressure within it so that the rate of formation of tissue fluid is slowed and at the same time the action of the muscle pump in propelling fluid from the extremity is aided. Elastic stockings should be made specially for the patient, as it is seldom that the contour of a lymphedematous leg can be fitted a stock size. The stockings used should be fashioned to fit the patient's leg when the volume of fluid in it is at a minimum, that is that the leg should be measured first thing in the morning, or even after a period of active dispersal of the edema as described below. The patient is likely to resent the wearing of an "ugly stocking"; tact and sympathy are required to convey that the lymphedematous leg has an abnormal appearance and is liable to become more abnormal if the elastic stocking is discarded. The stockings or stockings should be worn whenever the patient is up and about. Elastic or Ace bandages are less satisfactory because it is difficult for the patient to wrap them to achieve pressure of 50 mm. Hg at the ankle diminishing to 20 mm. Hg at the thigh. Moreover, even when snugly wrapped an elastic bandage tends to be more bulky than an elastic stocking.

Sometimes a decided effort to reduce the amount of swelling of the leg may seem desirable, for this purpose the patient is put to bed with the leg elevated. During this time dispersal of edema may be accelerated by use of a pneumatic device. The one most frequently used consists of inflatable legging or armlet which is placed on the limb and connected to an air pump which can provide a period of controlled pressure on the limb and a period when the limb is free of pressure. Satisfactory times and pressures are 45 seconds compression at 90 to 120 mm. Hg and 15 seconds release. Slightly more effective in reducing the size of the limb is an apparatus which consists of a series of eight overlapping inflatable bands on the limb. They are inflated in sequence so that pressure is first applied over the foot; then foot and ankle; foot, ankle, and lower calf and so on so that a wave of external pressure passes up the limb. After 15 seconds respite the cycle restarts. These devices are to be found in most physiotherapy departments, and they may also be bought or rented for use at home. A warning must be given that these devices should not be used if the possibility of infection of the limb exists for fear of disseminating the inflammatory agent.

Prevention of inflammation is important and is described in the section in this chapter on recurrent lymphangiitis. When skin breaks occur and become infected the condition is best treated in hospital with daily cleansing of the infected area, bathing of the leg in whirlpool baths and elevation of the limb so that the exudating areas can dry. Applications of 0.5 per cent silver nitrate solution control infection but have the disadvantage of permanent soilage of bed linen. Antibiotics should be used with caution because of the danger of inducing an allergic response.

Surgical treatment is reserved for patients with grosser forms of the disease and marked deformity. The measures taken are intended either to improve lymph drainage by providing channels for the lymph to drain through, or to excise the lymphedematous tissue. In the past operations were devised to bridge an interruption in lymph drainage by insertion of silk threads subcutaneously, or to bridge the edematous area to normal skin by means of pedicle grafts. The effectiveness of these procedures is difficult to judge because their performance coincides with an intensive course of other measures designed to reduce the edema. It is significant that this relatively simple form of treatment is hardly used at the present time.

Realization that anastomoses normally exist between the lymphatic channels and the veins led to the hope that drainage of an obstructed lymphatic trunk could be improved by anastomosing the trunk to an adjacent vein. So far this procedure has not proved successful. Somewhat more successful, by report, has been an extensive intra-abdominal operation to mobilize the omentum and bring it down to be implanted in the thigh. This operation must be regarded as still experimental and would seem to have a chance of success only when the lymphatics are competent but obstructed at the groin.

Excision of lymphedematous tissue is often referred to as the Kondoleon operation, though the procedure usually done is modified from that described by Charles or Homans. Skin flaps are lifted and the hyperemic lymphedematous tissue underlying them excised. The flaps are then used as skin grafts over the underlying deep tissues. The cosmetic results of these operations are less than satisfactory and should be reserved for limbs showing intolerable deformity. Elastic support of the leg is still required following these operations (Figs. 11-2 and 11-3)

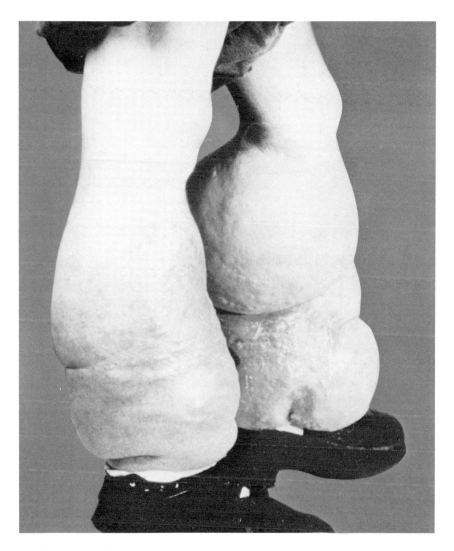

Fig. 11-2. Gross lymphedema of both legs beyond the knees. The skin shows eczematous and weeping eruption.

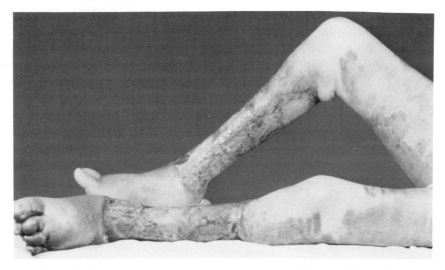

Fig. 11-3. Appearance of legs shown in Figure 11-2 after Kondoleon operation.

Secondary Lymphedema

The most frequent type of secondary lymphedema is that of the upper limb following radical mastectomy. The degree of swelling is seldom as severe as that seen in primary lymphedema being limited often to a puffiness of the hand. The onset occurs at different times after the operation, usually when the patient resumes activity but sometimes the appearance is delayed for months or years. Other causes of secondary lymphedema are listed in Table 11-1.

Treatment. The use of diuretics may help to limit the degree of swelling, but in cases where the discomfort and deformity of the arm limits social activity in the evening, the use of a pneumatic device for an hour in the late afternoon has proved beneficial.

The lymphedematous arm is liable to infection through minor injuries to the skin; these are treated as described under lymphangiitis. The patient should learn to protect the affected hand as a surgeon does his with scrupulous cleanliness, immediate attention to minor injuries, and avoidance of trauma by the use of gloves or a barrier cream.

TUMORS OF LYMPH VESSELS

Tumors of lymph vessels are seldom seen. They are comparable to tumors of blood vessels. The original classification of Wegner is the simplest though it has to be modified in individual cases.

Simple lymphangioma is almost always present from birth. The lesions are small and circumscribed with little tendency to grow. Occasionally excision is advisable for cosmetic reasons.

Cavernous lymphangiomata are also present from birth. The angioma is seldom only of lymph vessels, and the affected sinuses are usually filled with a mixture of blood and lymph. The tumor has a tendency to slow growth. If feasible the preferred treatment is surgical excision, though recurrence is common if the tumor cannot be completely excised. Even with satisfactory excision unsightly scars and wound infections are common. Radiotherapy may be of value.

Cystic hygroma is also usually present from birth but slowly enlarges. The tumor is most often in the neck and consists of a thin walled cystic mass containing serous fluid or lymph. It transilluminates well, which distinguishes it from a cyst of the branchial cleft. The cyst is liable to infection, and early excision is desirable though some surgeons have reported a high mortality. The tumor is resistant to radiotherapy.

REFERENCES

Heredity

Benson, P.F., Taylor, A.I., Gough, M.H.: Chromosome anomalies in primary lymphoedema. Lancet, *1*:461, 1967.

Esterly, J.R.: Congenital hereditary lymphoedema. J. Med. Genet., *2*:93, 1965.

Milroy, W.F.: Chronic heredity edema; Milroy's disease. JAMA, *91*:1172, 1928.

Patterson, D.F., Medway, W., Luginbuhl, H., and Chacko, S.: Congenital hereditary lymphoedema in the dog. Parts I & II. J. Med. Genet., *4*:145, 1967.

Lymphangiography

Kinmonth, J.B., Taylor, G.W., Tracey, G.D., and Marsh, J.D.: Primary lymphoedema; clinical and lymphangiographic studies of a series of 107 patients in which the lower limbs were affected. Brit. J. Surg., *45*:1, 1957.

Treatment

Babb, R.R., Spittell, J.A., Martin, W.J., and Schirger, A.: Prophylaxis of recurrent lymphangeitis complicating lymphedema. JAMA, *195*:871, 1966.

Homans, J.: Treatment of elephantiasis of the legs: a preliminary report. New Eng. J. Med., *215*:1099, 1936.

Kondoleon, E.: Die Lymphableitung, als Heilmittel bei chronischen Oedemen nach Quetschung. Munchen. Med. Wschr, *1*:525, 1912.

Sanderson, R.G., Fletcher, W.S: Conservative management of primary lymphedema. Northwest Med., *64*:584, 1965.

Filariasis

Colwell, E.J., Armstrong, D.R., Brown, J.D., et al.: Epidemiologic and serologic investigations of filariasis in indigenous populations and American soldiers in Vietnam. Amer. J. Trop. Med., *19*:227, 1970.

Sasa, M.: Microfilaria survey methods and analysis of survey data in filariasis control programmes. Bull. WHO, *37*:629, 1967.

Sawada, T., Sato, S., Matsuyama, S., Miuagi, H., Shimzato, J.: Intradermal skin test with antigen F.S.T. (FSCDI) on individuals in endemic areas. Japa. J. Exp. Med., *38*:405, 1968.

Tumors

Wegner, G.: Ueber lymphangiome. Arch. f. Klin. Chir., *20*:641, 1877.

Index